# SpringerBriefs in Well-Being and Quality of Life Research

More information about this series at http://www.springer.com/series/10150

Andrew J. Howell · Denise J. Larsen

# Understanding Other-Oriented Hope

## An Integral Concept Within Hope Studies

Springer

Andrew J. Howell
Department of Psychology
MacEwan University
Edmonton, AB
Canada

Denise J. Larsen
Department of Educational Psychology
University of Alberta
Edmonton, AB
Canada

ISSN 2211-7644 ISSN 2211-7652 (electronic)
SpringerBriefs in Well-Being and Quality of Life Research
ISBN 978-3-319-15006-2 ISBN 978-3-319-15007-9 (eBook)
DOI 10.1007/978-3-319-15007-9

Library of Congress Control Number: 2015930094

Springer Cham Heidelberg New York Dordrecht London


Springer International Publishing AG Switzerland is part of Springer Science+Business Media (www.springer.com)

# Contents

# Chapter 1
# Introduction to Other-Oriented Hope

## 1.1 General

*If our wives could see us now! I do hope they are better off in their camps and don't know what is happening to us.*
—Viktor Frankl, *Man's search for meaning,* 1992, p. 48.

Appearing in a book renowned for its compelling illustration of the life-sustaining and life-transforming process of maintaining hope and discovering meaning within the direst of circumstances, this statement by a concentration camp inmate and friend of Frankl reveals the potential importance of another, distinct psychological asset: hope directed not to one's own good fortune but rather to the good fortunes of others. Indeed, this example reveals several potentially important aspects of what we term *other-oriented hope*: First, the prisoner's expression of hope for the comfort of his spouse and those of his comrades suggests that other-oriented hope concerns those with whom we feel a connection, including those very close to us and those more remotely associated with us; thus, *degree of relationship* may be pertinent to other-oriented hope. Second, the expression of hope is directed toward both the spouses' well-being, on the one hand, and their lack of awareness of the plight of their husbands, on the other; thus, other-oriented hope has *approach and avoidance qualities*. Third, the example illustrates that hope held for others can be independent of whether one is able to exert an influence on desired outcomes; thus, other-oriented hope may involve relatively *low controllability*. Fourth, other-oriented hope, in this instance, surrounds desired outcomes of relatively low likelihood (i.e., given the imprisonment of the spouses); thus, this form of hope concerns outcomes that are *possible even if improbable*. Fifth, hoped-for events are separated in time or, as in this case, in space from the hopeful individual; thus, other-oriented hope is characterized by a *future time orientation* or, more generally, by *uncertainty*. Sixth, other-oriented hope may facilitate commitment on behalf of the inmate to persevere in his own circumstances, reflecting in part a desire to bear witness to potential realization of other-oriented hope; thus, other-oriented hope may induce a *general*



A.J. Howell and D.J. Larsen, *Understanding Other-Oriented Hope*,
SpringerBriefs in Well-Being and Quality of Life Research,
DOI 10.1007/978-3-319-15007-9_1

*motivated state* of engagement or vitality. Finally, the example is an instance of hope directed toward others despite catastrophic conditions experienced by the inmate; thus, other-oriented hope may often be a *response to adversity*, including adversity of both the hoping individual and those who are the targets of such hope. The fact that even the most imperiling personal circumstances do not preclude other-oriented hope suggests that this form of hope, too, springs eternal.

This monograph introduces, defines, exemplifies, and characterizes hope that is directed toward others rather than toward the self. In Chap. 2, we conceptualize other-oriented hope (or, synonymously, *vicarious hope*) as an aspect of the higher-order concept of *other-interest*. Building directly upon definitions and characteristics of self-oriented hope identified by past researchers and theorists, in Chap. 3 we construct a definition of other-oriented hope (*future-oriented belief, desire, and mental imagining surrounding a valued outcome of another person that is uncertain but possible*) and we identify various of its characteristics (e.g., future-orientation involving uncertainty). In Chap. 4, we review domains in which other-oriented hope has emerged in the research literature, and provide numerous examples of such empirically documented vicarious hope. These domains include hope held by parents of ill children, by informal caregivers, by professional caregivers, by teachers, and by individuals experiencing terminal illnesses; we also consider more general instances of other-oriented hope. We then strive, in Chap. 5, to understand other-oriented hope within theoretical frameworks emphasizing other-interest, self-transcendence, mental balance, and ecosystem versus egosystem motivational orientations. In Chap. 6, we address the fact that vicarious hope is likely to be associated with, and to require differentiation from, related concepts of compassion, empathy, love, caring, and worry. We argue that each of these, along with other-oriented hope, can be viewed as a constituent of the broader concept of other-interest. In our final Chap. 7, we examine several outstanding issues surrounding other-oriented hope (e.g., whether other strengths of character may manifest in a manner expressive of other-interest; the basis in realism of other-oriented hope); moreover, we identify ways in which other-oriented hope might be leveraged intentionally, such as in therapeutic situations, and we offer suggestions for the numerous directions which could be taken in future quantitative and qualitative research on other-oriented hope. Throughout, we employ examples of vicarious hope taken from research, clinical settings, and the authors' personal experiences in order to illustrate and apply other-oriented hope within real-life contexts. Throughout, we also critique the strengths and shortcomings of the available theory and research on other-oriented hope.

The study of hope has received significant attention from theorists, researchers, and practitioners over the past 50 years (Eliott 2005), some of it spurred on by, and indeed spurring on, the emergence of the field of positive psychology, or the *science of well-being*. A conceptual limitation of much (but by no means all) theorizing and research on hope is that, unlike Frankl's poignant example, it largely ignores other-oriented hope, instead casting hope in a singularly self-interested light. As an example, Snyder's (1994, 2002) highly influential and generative goal theory of hope conceptualizes hope as involving two key cognitive appraisals:

*Agency thinking* is the belief that one is capable of executing the means to attain desired ends, whereas *pathways thinking* is the belief that one is capable of generating those means (i.e., the 'will' and the 'ways' of hope, respectively). Although it has been suggested that Snyder's theory is incompatible with the idea of other-oriented hope (Bruininks and Malle 2005), nothing in these appraisals suggests that the desired goals toward which one is hopeful could not concern others in addition to, or indeed instead of, the self. Indeed, Snyder and Feldman (2000) discuss drawbacks of uniformly self-focused hope, stating:

> "There must be limits in the degree to which individuals pursue their personal goals .... If our most rewarded goals continue to involve status and the acquisition of money, many individuals may pursue these goals to the comparative detriment of other people. Hope, in this context, may fuel the individual's pursuit of egocentric goals, yet contribute to an inattention to the have-nots in society" (p. 410).

Snyder and Feldman (2000) also discuss the importance of the pursuit of collective goals; that is, goals reflecting shared or common aims of many within a group or society. Nonetheless, while recognizing the limits of self-focused hope and the possible importance of shared hope, other-oriented hope per se typically goes unrecognized in the literature on Snyder's goal theory of hope. Moreover, the goals studied by hope researchers operating from the perspective of Snyder's goal theory tend to be self-oriented ones, such as students' strivings to meet their own athletic and academic goals (Curry et al. 1997; Feldman and Dreher 2012). And, items on hope measures reflecting the theory are most readily interpreted as self-oriented (e.g., "There are lots of ways around any problem that I am facing now"; Snyder et al., 1996). Just as the dominant, fruitful, and well-supported hope theory of Snyder has afforded limited attention to other-oriented hope, so has the field of hope studies more generally.

In contradistinction to the more typical focus upon self-oriented hope, contemporary hope theorists have, on occasion, explicitly contrasted self-focused forms of hope with instances of hope directed toward others. According to Day (1969), the phrase 'hoping that' can be directed toward the self or others (e.g., *I hope that my brother passes his exam*), whereas the phrase 'hoping to' is self-directed (e.g., *I hope to get several chores done today*). Gottschalk's (1974) scheme for coding hope content from brief verbal samples gives equal weight to hope expressed toward others as to hope expressed toward the self. Godfrey (1987), in his integration of various philosophical views toward hope, distinguishes between hope aimed at one's own benefit (*hope-for-me*), hope aimed at another's benefit (*hope-for-another*), and hope aimed at a relationship with another (*shared life*, or *hope-for-us*). Hinds (1988) and Hendricks-Ferguson (1997) both note that a positive outlook for self *or others* is a critical attribute of hope among ill adolescents. McGeer (2004) contrasts egocentric hope with hope that instead reflects "alterocentric concerns of care" (p. 123). Wong and Heriot (2007) use the term *vicarious hope* in the context of parental hope held for ill children. Haase et al. (1992) identify *toward others* and *toward self* as two forms of goal orientation characterizing hope. Similarly, Eliott and Olver (2002) identify *focused on the self* versus *focused on another* as an important dualism within the study of hope. Finally, De Pretto et al. (2011) distinguish between personal hope, relational hope, and social hope, with the latter two forms of hope described as including *hopes for good things for significant others* and *hopes for good things for unrelated others*, respectively. Like positive psychology more generally, the study of hope stands to benefit from attempts to consider a greater focus upon others (Wong 2011).

Because vicarious hope remains a relatively neglected topic within hope theory and research, the current work aims to provide, for the first time, a robust conceptualization of other-oriented hope, and to review and critically examine existing literature on other-oriented hope. Constructs superficially resembling other-oriented hope but differentiable from it are not included herein. For example, although many theorists and researchers have commented upon the *relational* or *social* aspects of hope (e.g., Godfrey 1987; Snyder and Feldman 2000), that term typically does not refer to hope held by one person for another, but rather to the more general phenomena of one's hope being shaped by the hope of others, shared or collective hope, the achievement of one's goals depending upon the support of others, hoping that one will be accepted by others, or hope directed toward good relationships with others. On other occasions, hope is characterized in a manner which conflates self- and other-oriented aspects, blurring the status of such hope as other-oriented. We restrict our focus upon instances of hope held regarding the outcomes of another person when we employ the term *other-oriented hope*.

This treatise reviews both quantitative and qualitative research on hope and other-oriented hope. This inclusiveness reflects two generative traditions in hope research (Eliott 2005): quantitative research often conceptualizes hope as a unidimensional concept and focuses upon scale development and establishing generalized correlates of hope (i.e., focusing on differences in hope *between persons* and the correlates of those differences), whereas qualitative research typically conceptualizes hope as multidimensional in nature, and concerns hope as a lived experience and the application of hope to contexts such as medicine (i.e., focusing on hope *within persons* and the unique experience of a particular individual's hope in real-life settings). Both traditions yield data and theoretical insights in support of other-oriented hope. Moreover, investigations that yield some of the strongest evidence in support of other-oriented hope are those that combine quantitative and qualitative methods (i.e., mixed-methods research such as that by Averill et al. 1990 and by Herth 1990, 1993). Finally, the quantitative and qualitative research reviewed herein is multidisciplinary in nature; the empirical review draws upon the work of researchers within the academic disciplines of nursing, medicine, social work, psychology, counselling, and others.

With this brief introduction to other-oriented hope, we next provide a framework for understanding the place and role of hope that is directed toward others. Specifically, in Chap. 2, we examine the idea of *other-interest* and position other-oriented hope within this psychological dimension.

But first, let's consider an example of other-oriented hope:

**Box 1.1: Other-Oriented Hope and Suicide**
I (A. H.) recall my own experience of other-oriented hope in relation to the publicized suicide of a 19 year-old undergraduate psychology student in Edmonton, Alberta, in February 2014. According to news reports, the man, who experienced bullying as a youth in relation to having epilepsy, jumped in front of a commuter train. Adding to the tragedy, another teen, a young woman, stole the deceased man's backpack from the train platform after witnessing the man's death. The discordant image of one tortured soul taking his life and, unmoved, another taking the dead man's backpack was massively unsettling.

Imagining the man as a student in one of my own psychology courses, I recall a profound feeling of regret over the man's lack of hope, revealing an underlying form of other-oriented hope, a kind of *hope that another might have hope*. Such other-oriented hope is also revealed in societal-wide suicide prevention tactics, such as signage on bridges stating, "There is always hope. Call the Distress Line", shorthand for "We hope that you will find the hope you need to get through these extremely challenging times, and we want to help" or, based on Jevne (2005), "We hope that you can envision a future in which you want to participate".

I also experienced other-oriented hope toward the young woman, hope that she would see the error in her ways, experience compassion for the deceased man and his loved ones, and return the backpack to the family. Behind such hope was empathy for the woman's dire personal circumstances, including substance dependence, and the belief that the woman could redeem herself and start a new, more hopeful, life if she could face-up to her transgression. Indeed, within a few days of the tragedy, the young woman and her family returned the backpack to the grieving relatives, who responded with appreciation and forgiveness. I experienced my own heightened hope as a result of the woman making amends for her wrongdoing in honour of the deceased individual and the family responding with such compassion of their own. Importantly, the young man's journal, contained within the backpack, confirmed that his death was a suicide. Said his stepfather, "He was overwhelmed by so many things and he just wanted peace. We hope he finds it now" (Edmonton Sun, February 2014). Poignantly, the family's hope toward their son persisted even beyond his death.

## References

Averill, J. R., Catlin, G., & Chon, K. K. (1990). *Rules of hope*. New York: Springer.
Bruininks, P., & Malle, B. F. (2005). Distinguishing hope from optimism and related affective states. *Motivation and Emotion, 29*, 327–355.

Curry, L. A., Snyder, C. R., Cook, D. L., Ruby, D. C., & Rehm, M. (1997). Role of hope in academic and sport achievement. *Journal of Personality and Social Psychology, 73*, 1257–1267.

Day, J. P. (1969). Hope. *American Philosophical Quarterly, 6*, 89–102.

De Pretto, L., King, R. B., Shin, S.-H., & Simpson, A. (2011). *What does hope mean to people? Cross-national analysis of the lay construct of hope.* Paper presented at the 9th Biennial Conference of the Asian Association of Social Psychology.

Eliott, J. A. (2005). What have we done with hope? A brief history. In J. A. Eliott (Ed.), *Interdisciplinary perspectives on hope* (pp. 3–45). New York: Nova Science Publishers.

Eliott, J. A., & Olver, I. N. (2002). The discursive properties of "hope": A qualitative analysis of cancer patients' speech. *Qualitative Health Research, 12*, 173–193.

Feldman, D. B., & Dreher, D. E. (2012). Can hope be changed in 90 minutes? Testing the efficacy of a single-session goal-pursuit intervention for college students. *Journal of Happiness Studies, 13*, 745–759.

Frankl, V. E. (1992). *Man's search for meaning: An introduction to logotherapy* (4th ed.). Boston: Beacon Press.

Godfrey, J. J. (1987). *A philosophy of human hope*. Dordrecht: Martinus Nijhoff Publishers.

Gottschalk, L. A. (1974). A hope scale applicable to verbal samples. *Archives of General Psychiatry, 30*, 779–785.

Haase, J. E., Britt, T., Coward, D. D., Kline Leidy, N., & Penn, P. E. (1992). Simultaneous concept analysis of spiritual perspective, hope, acceptance and self-transcendence. *Journal of Nursing Scholarship, 24*, 141–147.

Hendricks-Ferguson, V. L. (1997). An analysis of the concept of hope in the adolescent with cancer. *Journal of Pediatric Oncology Nursing, 14*, 73–80.

Herth, K. (1990). Fostering hope in terminally-ill people. *Journal of Advanced Nursing, 13*, 1250–1259.

Herth, K. (1993). Hope in older adults in community and institutional settings. *Issues in Mental Health Nursing, 14*, 139–156.

Hinds, P. S. (1988). Adolescent hopefulness in illness and health. *Advances in Nursing Science, 10*, 79–88.

Jevne, R. F. (2005). Hope: The simplicity and complexity. In J. Eliott (Ed.), *Interdisciplinary perspectives on hope* (pp. 259–289). Hauppauge, New York: Nova Science.

McGeer, V. (2004). The art of good hope. *Annals of the American Academy of Political and Social Science, 592*, 100–127.

Snyder, C. R. (1994). *The psychology of hope: You can get there from here*. New York: Free Press.

Snyder, C. R. (2002). Hope theory: Rainbows in the mind. *Psychological Inquiry, 13*, 1047–1084.

Snyder, C. R., & Feldman, D. B. (2000). Hope for the many: An empowering social agenda. In C. R. Snyder (Ed.), *Handbook of hope: Theory, measures, and applications* (pp. 389–412). New York: Academic Press.

Snyder, C. R., Sympson, S. C., Ybasco, F. C., Borders, T. F., Babyak, M. A., & Higgins, R. L. (1996). Development and validation of the State Hope Scale. *Journal of Personality and Social Psychology, 70*, 321–335.

Wong, M. G., & Heriot, S. A. (2007). Vicarious futurity in autism and childhood dementia. *Journal of Autism and Developmental Disorders, 37*, 1833–1841.

Wong, P. T. P. (2011). Positive psychology 2.0: Towards a balanced interactive model of the good life. *Canadian Psychology, 52*, 69–81.

# Chapter 2
# Other-Oriented Hope Reflects an Orientation Toward Others

## 2.1 General

> *Every motive or act falls somewhere on a spectrum between extreme selfishness and extreme unselfishness, depending on the relative weight we give our own interests and the interests of others.*
> —Jencks 1990, p. 53

In Chap. 1, we underscored the fact that the field of hope studies has given limited attention to hope that is directed toward others. The field's lack of focus upon other-oriented hope reflects, in part, the fact that much research and theorizing has concerned the *process* of hoping more than the *content* of hopes, that is, the nature of hoped-for outcomes or events. For example, Snyder's (2002) goal theory of hope emphasizes the types of cognitions that hopeful individuals manifest, including agency thinking and pathways thinking. Although such thinking processes are ultimately aimed at the attainment of specific goals or outcomes, those outcomes are oftentimes not considered to be of foremost concern. Rather, the act of hoping or the process of being hopeful is deemed most important (i.e., the characteristics and adaptive benefits of being a hopeful person), while the objects of a person's hopes may remain unspecified. At other times, the content of hoped-for-outcomes is constrained by the research context, as in the case of students being asked directly about their hope regarding their academic lives. Nonetheless, enough research concerning the content of people's hope has been conducted to permit an evaluation of the nature of hope vis a vis its self- and other-oriented nature, a topic which we pursue in detail in Chap. 4. In the current chapter, we consider several reasons why we would expect the content of people's hope, upon systematic evaluation, to occasionally or even frequently concern others.



A.J. Howell and D.J. Larsen, *Understanding Other-Oriented Hope*,
SpringerBriefs in Well-Being and Quality of Life Research,
DOI 10.1007/978-3-319-15007-9_2

## 2.2 Psychological Concepts Pertinent to Other-Oriented Hope

There are several well-established psychological concepts that are congruent with the idea that our hopes may often be directed toward the well-being of others. Although the literature on these concepts rarely alludes to hope or, rarer still, to other-oriented hope, we view these concepts as highly congenial with the assertion that the content of hope will not infrequently concern others. These include the concepts of social interest, belongingness, relatedness, social value orientation, the prosocial personality, communion, self-transcendent values, and altruism.

Adler's (1938) concept of *social interest* provides reason to anticipate that hope may frequently be directed toward the well-being of others. Social interest is defined as having "interests in the interests of another" (Ansbacher 1991, p. 37). As described by Leak and Leak (2006):

> Social interest, or Gemeinschaftsgefuhl, involves a sense of social feeling toward all humankind, and the essence of social interest is the valuing of something outside the self without ulterior motives: a true absence of self-centeredness, egocentricity, and self-absorption. Social interest is based on one's identification with others and a transcendence of self-interest that results in a genuine concern with and striving for community and human welfare. (p. 208)

Crandall (1980) emphasizes that social interest supplements, rather than contradicts or opposes, self-interest. According to Crandall, social interest influences "a person's attention, perception, thinking about others, feeling such as empathy and sympathy, and finally motives and overt behavior relating to cooperation, helping, sharing, contributing, and so on" (p. 481).

**Box 2.1: Hoping and Helping**

Regan Holt is an experienced inner-city junior high school teacher. She has long infused her curriculum with an intentional and explicit hope focus, believing that this provides vital life learning and an invaluable classroom resource. She tells a story that invites us to consider the connections between social interest and other-oriented hope. An advocate for her students, she also challenges common social conceptions of youth who grow up in challenged neighbourhoods.

Ms. Holt remembers early in her career taking her class on a walking field trip. They were headed to an activity that had been planned during a class discussion on how the students could offer hope to their community. As the class filed out the school and down the steps of the old brick building, they passed a homeless man slouched by the hand-railing and begging for money. Recognizing a potential incident in the making, Ms. Holt watched, ready to intervene as needed. Rather than a confrontation, she witnessed several of the students stop briefly to give the man loose change as they offered words of concern for his welfare.

Research supports the psychological benefits of expressing social interest. Crandall (1980) demonstrated that social interest is associated with several indices of well-being, such as greater purpose in life and lower physical stress. Leak and Leak (2006) showed, in a first study, that scores on the Social Interest Index positively correlated with a number of markers of adaptive psychological functioning, such as positive affect, satisfaction with life, vitality, and an intrinsic value orientation. In a second study, they showed that social interest positively correlated with measures of prosocial tendencies (e.g., being empathic) and prosocial moral reasoning (e.g., empathic-internalized moral reasoning). Interestingly, Barlow et al. (2009) showed that hope was a specific correlate of social interest.

Social interest resembles a more recently studied social psychological construct, that of *belongingness* (Ansbacher 1991). Baumeister and Leary (1995) argue that humans have a fundamental need to belong with others, a need viewed as innate and universal and as evolving because of the survival and reproductive advantages of cooperative and collective living. Baumeister and Leary identify two key features of the need for belongingness: people have a need for frequent positive interactions with others, and people have a need for relationships of ongoing and mutual affective concern.

Baumeister and Leary (1995) go on to identify several lines of evidence consistent with viewing belongingness as a fundamental human need, such as evidence that we form bonds with others readily and we break them only reluctantly. A further line of evidence supportive of the belongingness hypothesis, one most pertinent to the current context, is that the need for belongingness has significant effects on cognition, or thinking processes, and hence possibly on the content of people's hope. Baumeister and Leary review evidence that a significant amount of cognitive processing is devoted to our interactions and relationships; that self-serving biases in our cognitive processing are often extended to close others; that our optimism often 'spills over' to colour our views of close others' futures; that we at times selectively forget undesirable behaviours committed by those close to us; and that, in general, our explanations for events often emphasize interpersonal as opposed to impersonal causes. In other words, much of our thinking life revolves around others, and much of the favourable thinking we engage in about ourselves is generalized to those with whom we have relationships. As stated by Baumeister and Leary, "Concern with belongingness appears to be a powerful factor shaping human thought" (p. 505). While no research on hope was included by Baumeister and Leary in advancing their belongingness hypothesis (indeed, very limited research on hope was available at the time), it is nonetheless a logical extension of their view to argue that one's hope should reflect concern toward others in a manner similar to one's causal attributions or one's memories. That is, if human thought is shaped by our concern for belongingness, so too should human hoping, as hoping is, at least in part, future-oriented thought.

The concept of *attachment* is also pertinent to the notion of other-oriented hope. Bowlby (1969) argues for the importance of establishing a secure attachment with others when it comes to developing adaptive emotional regulation and coping strategies. Positive relationship experiences during infancy allow for the proper development of socio-emotional skills, and for positive representations of relationships that are carried forward to new experiences, including the later ability to provide care to one's own offspring. Mikulincer and Shaver (2012) review evidence that securely attached individuals also develop a greater sense of interest in caring for the well-being of others. In an earlier pronouncement of this viewpoint, Mikulincer et al. (2003) state that:

> On the one hand, persons who hold a chronic sense of secure base or persons whose sense of secure base is contextually activated in a specific situation would have more available resources to attend to others' needs and to provide adequate help and care…On the other hand, doubts about having a secure base may inhibit concern for others' welfare. Insecurely attached persons may be so egoistically self-focused on their own attachment needs and distress that they may lack the necessary resources to attend to others' needs and to engage in caring behaviors. (p. 301)

In a series of studies, Mikulincer et al. (2003) found support for these hypotheses; for example, they showed that priming a secure attachment base increased the endorsement of universalism and benevolence values, that is, values considered to transcend the self in their focus upon others (see below).

Another important theoretical advance is the work of Bakan (1966), who distinguishes between *agency* and *communion* as two key life orientations. Agency describes a drive to manage one's environment with efficacy, whereas communion describes a drive to befriend and care for others. Cislak and Wojciszke (2008) argue that agentic qualities are associated with self-interest, whereas communal qualities are associated with other-interest:

> Communal properties are other-profitable because other people…directly benefit from such traits like kindness, helpfulness, or honesty and are harmed by their opposites…In the same vein, agentic qualities are self-profitable because they are immediately rewarding for the acting person: whatever one does, it is better for him or her to do it efficiently. (p. 1104)

Cislak and Wojciszke (2008) showed that when behaviour is perceived as serving self-interests, inferences of agency are derived, whereas when behaviour is perceived as serving other-interests, inferences of communion are derived.

In a similar vein, Abele and Wojciszke (in press) argue that the two major dimensions underlying social cognition are communion and agency, wherein communion concerns relationships and group functioning whereas agency concerns competence and task completion. These dimensions are conceptualized as being independent of each other. This model is congenial with the idea that hope content could reflect either agency or communion and therefore be relatively self-oriented or other-oriented, respectively.

There is emerging support for a relationship between communion and hope, including other-oriented hope. In recent research, Larsen et al. (2014) examined client experiences in hope-focused group treatment for people with chronic pain. Employing qualitative methods, a key category in the findings was entitled *communion,* and was comprised of themes related to group members experiencing (a) creation of community, (b) support from others, and (c) hope for others.

Hope for others included both hope for specific hoped-for objects for another (such as an upcoming trip the other had planned) and hope that other group members could find hope itself.

Another theoretical concept of potential relevance to the notion of other-oriented hope comes from the theory of self-determination (e.g., Deci and Ryan 2000; Ryan and Deci 2001). According to this view, the key psychological needs that humans require to be met in order to experience well-being are the need for autonomy (or, self-governance), the need for competence (or, self-efficacy), and the need for relatedness. *Relatedness*, similar to belongingness, concerns humans' inherent proclivity to forge meaningful, supportive relationships with others. To the extent that this need (in conjunction with the remaining two) is well-met, individuals will grow and flourish in their lives. To the extent that this need (in conjunction with the remaining two) goes unmet, individuals' thriving will be impeded.

Self-determination theory argues that these psychological needs can be met most directly through the pursuit of intrinsic aspirations, which are first-order or non-reducible aspirations that are inherently healthy for humans, such as affiliating with others and striving to improve one's community. Such aspirations can be contrasted with extrinsic aspirations, such as wealth, fame, or status, which are indirect, less efficient, and more problematic routes toward the meeting of psychological needs. If good relationships are key to our mental health, if others need our support and love to foster *their* well-being, and if good relationships can be facilitated through aspirations such as affiliating with others and contributing to a better social climate, then it is likely that the outcomes that we hope for on a day-to-day basis, and indeed our general outlook on the world, will frequently concern the welfare of others. So, although no research within self-determination theory has concerned the extent to which our hope refers to others' welfare, it is reasonable to suppose that directing our hope towards others will be a frequent experience.

Another concept associated with our relationship to others is *social value orientation*, a concept chiefly studied in the area of decision-making. As a counterpoint to the position that rational choices will always be directed toward the maximization of gains only for the self, social value orientation conceptualizes a range of individual preferences for decision making, including preferences for choices that are selfish or individualist, competitive, and prosocial (Bogaert et al. 2008). Bogaert et al. describe prosocial individuals as being willing to cooperate because they view cooperation as intelligent (as opposed to irrational) and of high moral standard. Research has shown that prosocial individuals cooperate more and are more sensitive to the impact of their behaviour on others (Bogaert et al. 2008). Also, research by Van Lange et al. (2007) showed that prosocial individuals make more donations, such as buying something for a good cause or donating used clothing. Moreover, whereas prosocial individuals were more likely to donate to third world organizations or to charity and societal organizations than either individualists or competitors, no differences occurred concerning donations to health organizations, church organizations, sport organizations or education organizations. This pattern suggests that prosocial individuals are characterized especially by their greater willingness to give to others under conditions in which they are unlikely to benefit directly and the recipient is unknown to them.

Interestingly, Murphy et al. (2011) present evidence that the prosocial response type, as assessed with three different measures of social value orientation, was the most common response type, characterizing 59 % of their sample of young adult Europeans. Research has also considered the origins of the prosocial orientation to decision-making. Van Lange et al. (1997) showed that prosocial individuals, relative to individualists and competitors, are more likely to evidence a secure adult attachment (e.g., finding it easy to trust and to get close to others) and that prosocial individuals are more likely to have a greater number of siblings, more older siblings, and more female siblings than individualists and competitors.

Prosociality has also been considered by personality theorists. Penner et al. (1995) devised a measure of *prosocial personality* comprised of two factors: The first factor, other-oriented empathy, includes thoughts and feelings regarding the well-being of others. The second factor, helpfulness, concerns the tendency to be helpful toward others in one's behaviour. Caprara et al. (2012) showed that having a prosocial disposition is associated with the personality trait of agreeableness, with self-transcendent values of universalism and benevolence, and with self-efficacy beliefs concerning the ability to be attuned to others' emotional experiences.

Caprara et al.'s (2012) finding of a role for self-transcendent values in prosociality is conceptually related to Schwartz's (1994) model of human values and the relevance of a subset of those values to the tendency to take into account the concerns of others (see also Schwartz 2010). Schwartz identifies 10 universal human values: universalism, benevolence, conformity, tradition, security, power, achievement, hedonism, stimulation, and self-direction. These values are placed (in the order listed) within a circumplex (circular) arrangement, such that values adjacent to each other (e.g., power and achievement) are positively correlated, whereas those opposite each other (e.g., power and benevolence) are negatively correlated, or antagonistic. The values of universalism and benevolence are considered to be *self-transcendent* values, as they involve placing importance on the needs of others. Specifically, universalism involves concern directed toward all of humanity, such as viewing all people as equal, and benevolence involves concern directed toward close others. According to Schwartz (1994), people differ in the importance they place on each of the 10 value types. For example, some may place a great amount of importance on universalism and benevolence, whereas others may place very little importance on these values, but instead may place great importance on opposing, self-enhancing, values of achievement and power.

Keltner et al. (2014) recently reviewed the literature on prosociality, underscoring its basis in the nervous system, intrapersonal processes, interpersonal processes, group processes, and cultural values and norms. Falling clearly in favour of viewing humans as a prosocial species, they concluded that, "The study of prosocial behavior … has matured enough to produce general scholarly consensus that prosociality is widespread, intuitive, and rooted deeply within our biological makeup" (p. 425).

Addressing the issue of the motivation behind prosocial behaviour, Batson and Shaw (1991) argue cogently that some prosocial behaviour reflects *altruism*, defined as "a motivational state with the ultimate goal of increasing another's welfare" (p. 108). Egoism, in contrast, is concerned with increasing one's own welfare. Batson and Shaw review evidence in support of the role of empathic responding to another's plight in the instigation of altruistic behaviour toward others. For example, they show that among people high in empathy, but not among those low in empathy, being provided with the opportunity to escape the presence of a suffering individual (i.e., reflecting the egoistic motivation to reduce one's personal distress caused by exposure to a vulnerable other), does not reduce helping behaviour. Reflecting people's propensity for prosocial behaviour fueled by altruism, Batson and Shaw conclude that "Other people can be more to us than sources of information, stimulation, and reward … as we seek our own welfare. We have the potential to care about their welfare as well" (p. 120). The existence of prosocial personality traits or values, and of truly altruistic behaviour, is compatible with the occurrence of other-oriented hope.

A number of additional theoretical concepts which pit processes that are self-focused versus those that are other-focused can be seen to pertain to other-oriented hope; a few will be briefly mentioned here. Dunn et al. (2008) showed that giving away money to others has a bigger impact on well-being than spending it on ourselves. Brown et al. (2003) showed that providing support to others was associated with reduced mortality whereas receiving support from others was not. The concept of *life purpose* has been associated with attending to others, as in this definition of purpose by Damon et al. (2003): "A stable and generalized intention to accomplish something that is at once meaningful to the self and of consequence to the world beyond the self" (p. 121).

## 2.3 The Concepts of Self-Interest and Other-Interest

The theoretically and empirically-substantiated concepts of social interest, belongingness, communion, attachment, relatedness, social value orientation, prosociality, altruism, and universalism and benevolence values point to a strong proclivity among humans to orient toward the interests of others. The social psychologist Brewer (2004) argues that social living requires humans to achieve a *balance* between benefitting the self and benefitting others (see also Gerbasi and Prentice 2013; Korsgaard and Meglino 2008). Brewer states that "humans are not driven either by unmitigated individual selfishness or by noncontingent altruism, but instead show the capacity for variable motivation and behavior patterns contingent on the state of the environment" (p. 109). Similarly, MacIntyre (1999) underscores the notion that balancing self-directed and other-directed motives is integral to our social existence: "…we become neither self-rather-than-other-regarding nor other-rather-than-self-regarding, neither egoists nor altruists, but those whose passions and inclinations are directed to what is both our good and the good of others" (p. 160). And, Sternberg (2001) argues that wisdom, and thus wise living, is "not simply about maximizing one's own or someone else's self-interest, but about balancing various self-interests (intrapersonal) with the interests of others (interpersonal) and other aspects of the context in which one lives (extrapersonal), such as one's city or country or environment or even God" (p. 231).

Recently, Gerbasi and Prentice (2013) sought to conceptualize and quantify individual differences in self- and other-interest. They argue that self- and other-interest are relatively independent psychological dimensions underlying behaviour, that they operate in tandem with each other and, as a result, that any one behaviour may be motivated by a mix of both forms of interest. Gerbasi and Prentice define other-interest as a motivational orientation toward "the pursuit of gains for others in socially valued domains, including material goods, social status, recognition, academic or occupational achievement, and happiness" (p. 497). They characterize other-interest as varying between individuals and across situations. And, they allow that behaviour which pursues others' interests can itself reflect influences that are egoistic (e.g., reflecting one's inherent interdependence with others) and those that are altruistic (e.g., reflecting personality factors such as compassion). Gerbasi and Prentice operationalize the construct of other-interest with rating-scale items such as, *I am constantly looking for ways for my acquaintances to get ahead* and *I try to help my acquaintances by telling other people about their successes*.

In research validating their operationalization of other-interest, Gerbasi and Prentice (2013) showed that, relative to scores on a parallel measure of self-interest, other-interest scores were more positively associated with the endorsement of benevolence and universalism values. Other-interest scores were also associated with holding a conception of the self as interdependent with others. Conversely, other-interest scores were less positively correlated with achievement and power values and with materialistic leanings. In a subsequent study, the researchers showed that priming prosocial values led to an increase in other-interest scores. Finally, additional studies showed that other-interest scores predicted behaviour that was believed to benefit another person, and that other-interest scores predicted prosocial choices in a computer-based social dilemma game.

This recent work provides support for the distinction between psychological processes behind self-oriented thinking and behaviour and those behind other-oriented thinking and behaviour and, in so doing, provides an empirically-supported conceptual basis to the present attempt to distinguish between self- and other-oriented hope. Other-oriented hope is viewed herein as a specific manifestation of the more general psychological dimension termed other-interest. Other specific manifestations of other-interest would include a prosocial value orientation, the prosocial personality, the need for relatedness, the need for belongingness, and high social interest. Whereas other-interest encapsulates a broad and generalized orientation toward valuing, recognizing, facilitating, promoting, and celebrating positive outcomes for others that have occurred in the past or present, or that may occur in the future, other-oriented hope cleaves that portion of other-interest specific to the harbouring of future-oriented hope for others and (where possible) attendant strivings toward meeting those ends. Moreover, further differentiating other-oriented hope from the broader concept of other-interest are the unique attributes of other-oriented hope (to be outlined in Chap. 4), including relatively high uncertainty, low control, and low likelihood.

In summary, the social nature of humans means that we have both self- and other-interests, that we strive to find an optimal balance between these interests, and that people will differ in the degree to which they express each kind of interest, with those who show greater other-interest also behaving especially helpfully toward, and cooperating with, others. Other-oriented hope is viewed as a specific form of other-interest, one in which we reveal our interest in the welfare of others by apportioning some of our future-oriented mental imaginings to others' welfare in addition to our own, more self-focused, hope. In the next chapter, we examine the definition and characteristics of hope in both its self- and other-oriented manifestations.

**Box 2.2: Hope Reflects Many Interests**

Some time ago in my counselling psychology practice, I (D. L.) had the opportunity to work with a professional, Lensa, who had struggled with depression for many years. Her visit to my office was precipitated by several difficult circumstances. Her brother had recently been in serious trouble with the law, she described her workplace experiences via numerous examples of bullying, and a recent intimate relationship had collapsed. Lensa said that she sought therapy to learn that there was still hope. As I learned about her history and the painful experiences she had recently endured, I asked if she might craft a list of her hopes with me. She agreed and we began together. As we talked, her list began to grow. Lensa began with 'big' hopes like the hope to end world hunger, the hope to save child soldiers, and even the hope for global well-being—all other-oriented hopes. I said that I shared these hopes with her. We could both hope for these things together. Nevertheless, on clinical reflection, I was concerned about the broad scope and ambition of her hopes given her long standing struggle with depression. And so, I also reminded her that while some of our hopes can be large, some of our hopes can also be small, some can be serious, some can be fun, some can be short-term, some can be long-term, some can be likely, and some may be unlikely. As we talked, she began to add to her list. She hoped to see her son and his new young family next weekend. She hoped to take dance classes. She hoped her new granddaughter would one day learned to play the violin, and so on. As our session came to a close, we reviewed her hopes and found evidence that some hope still existed in her life and some of it was very likely to be realized. Indeed, she had plans to see her son's family on the weekend. We hadn't finished our work together but we had found a hopeful place to start. As a therapist, I held hope for Lensa, too.

## References

Abele, A. E., & Wojciszke, B. (in press). Communal and agentic content in social cognition: A dual perspective model. *Advances in Experimental Social Psychology.*

Adler, A. (1938). *Social interest: A challenge to mankind.* J. Linton & R. Vaughan (Trans.). London: Faber and Faber Ltd.

Ansbacher, H. L. (1991). The concept of social interest. *Individual Psychology, 47*, 28–46.

Bakan, D. (1966). *The duality of human existence.* Chicago: Rand McNally.

Barlow, P. J., Tobin, D. J., & Schmidt, M. M. (2009). Social interest and positive psychology: Positively aligned. *Journal of Individual Psychology, 65*, 192–202.

Batson, C. D., & Shaw, L. L. (1991). Evidence for altruism: Toward a pluralism of prosocial motives. *Psychological Inquiry, 2*, 107–122.

Baumeister, R. F., & Leary, M. R. (1995). The need to belong: Desire for interpersonal attachments as a fundamental human motivation. *Psychological Bulletin, 117*, 497–529.

Bogaert, S., Boone, C., & Declerck, C. (2008). Social value orientation and cooperation in social dilemmas: A review and conceptual model. *British Journal of Social Psychology, 47*, 453–480.

Bowlby, J. (1969). *Attachment and loss: Vol. 1. Attachment.* New York: Basic Books.

Brewer, M. B. (2004). Taking the social origins of human nature seriously: Toward a more imperialist social psychology. *Personality and Social Psychology Review, 8*, 107–113.

Brown, S. L., Nesse, R. M., Vinokur, A. D., & Smith, D. M. (2003). Providing social support may be more beneficial than receiving it: Results from a prospective study of mortality. *Psychological Science, 14*, 320–327.

Caprara, G. V., Alessandri, G., & Eisenberg, N. (2012). Prosociality: The contribution of traits, values, and self-efficacy beliefs. *Journal of Personality and Social Psychology, 102*, 1289–1303.

Cislak, A., & Wojciszke, B. (2008). Agency and communion are inferred from actions serving interests of self or others. *European Journal of Social Psychology, 38*, 1103–1110.

Crandall, J. E. (1980). Adler's concept of social interest: Theory, measurement, and implications for adjustment. *Journal of Personality and Social Psychology, 39*, 481–495.

Damon, W., Menon, J., & Bronk, K. C. (2003). The development of purpose during adolescence. *Applied Developmental Science, 7*, 119–128.

Deci, E. L., & Ryan, R. M. (2000). The "what" and "why" of goal pursuits: Human needs and the self-determination of behavior. *Psychological Inquiry, 11*, 227–268.

Dunn, E. W., Aknin, L. B., & Norton, N. I. (2008). Spending money on others promotes happiness. *Science, 319*, 1687–1688.

Gerbasi, M. E., & Prentice, D. A. (2013). The Self- and Other-Interest Inventory. *Journal of Personality and Social Psychology, 105*, 495–514.

Jencks, C. (1990). Varieties of altruism. In J. J. Mansbridge (Ed.), *Beyond self-interest* (pp. 54–67). Chicago: University of Chicago Press.

Keltner, D., Kogan, A., Piff, P. K., & Saturn, S. R. (2014). The sociocultural appraisals, values, and emotions (SAVE) framework of prosociality: Core processes from gene to meme. *Annual Review of Psychology, 65*, 425–460.

Korsgaard, M. A., & Meglino, B. (2008). Beyond the individualistic self: A framework for prosocial motives and judgments. In H. A. Wayment & J. J. Bauer (Eds.), *Transcending self-interest: Psychological explorations of the quiet ego* (pp. 183–195). Washington, DC: American Psychological Association.

Larsen, D., King, R., Stege, R., & Egeli, N. (2014). *Clients' experiences of hope in a hope strengths-based group activity for individuals with chronic pain.* Unpublished manuscript.

Leak, G. K., & Leak, K. C. (2006). Adlerian social interest and positive psychology: A conceptual and empirical integration. *Journal of Individual Psychology, 62*, 207–223.

MacIntyre, A. (1999). *Dependent rational animals: Why human beings need the virtues.* Chicago: Open Court Publishing.

Mikulincer, M., Gillath, O., Sapir-Lavid, Y., Yaakobi, E., Arias, K., Tal-Alonni, L., & Bor, G. (2003). Attachment theory and concern for others' welfare: Evidence that activation of the sense of secure base promotes endorsement of self-transcendent values. *Basic and Applied Social Psychology, 25*, 299–312.

Mikulincer, M., & Shaver, P. R. (2012). Adult attachment orientations and relationship processes. *Journal of Family Theory and Review, 4*, 259–274.

Murphy, R. O., Ackermann, K. A., & Handgraff, M. J. J. (2011). Measuring social value orientation. *Judgment and Decision Making, 6*, 771–781.

Penner, L. A., Fritzsche, B. A., Craiger, J. P., & Freifeld, T. S. (1995). Measuring the prosocial personality. In J. Butcher & C. D. Speilberger (Eds.), *Advances in personality assessment* (Vol. 10). Hillsdale, NJ: LEA.

Ryan, R. M., & Deci, E. L. (2001). On happiness and human potentials: A review of research on hedonic and eudaimonic well-being. *Annual Review of Psychology, 52*, 141–166.

Schwartz, S. (1994). Are there universal aspects in the structure and contents of human values? *Journal of Social Issues, 50*, 19–45.

Schwartz, S. H. (2010). Basic values: How they motivate and inhibit prosococial behavior. In M. Mikulincer & P. R. Shaver (Eds.), *Prosocial motives, emotions, and behavior: The better angels of our nature* (pp. 221–241). Washington, DC: American Psychological Association.

Snyder, C. R. (2002). Hope theory: Rainbows in the mind. *Psychological Inquiry, 13*, 1047–1084.

Sternberg, R. J. (2001). Why schools should teach for wisdom: The balance theory of wisdom in educational settings. *Educational Psychology, 36*, 227–245.

Van Lange, P. A. M., Bekkers, R., Schuyt, T. N. M., & Van Vugt, M. (2007). From games to giving: Social value orientation predicts donations to noble causes. *Basic and Applied Social Psychology, 29*, 375–384.

Van Lange, P. A. M., Otten, W., De Bruin, E. M. N., & Joireman, J. A. (1997). Development of prosocial, individualistic, and competitive orientations: Theory and preliminary evidence. *Journal of Personality and Social Psychology, 73*, 733–746.

# Chapter 3
# Definitions and Attributes of Hope, and Their Application to Other-Oriented Hope

## 3.1 General

> *We cannot hope well without taking a hopeful interest in the hopes of others and* vice versa.
> —McGeer 2004, p. 125

Hope is an oft-defined concept; here we examine four definitions, from various academic perspectives, that converge on central attributes of hope. We then present integrative definitions of hope and other-oriented hope. We examine evidence for the differentiation of hope from related states such as optimism and joy. We then examine numerous attempts to conceptualize hope from a multidimensional perspective, and extract those dimensions that are common or frequently occurring across such conceptualizations. Finally, we explore the relevance of those dimensions to other-oriented hope.

## 3.2 Definitions of Hope

Lazarus (1999), a psychologist, writes that to hope is "to believe that something positive, which does not presently apply to one's own life, could still materialize" (p. 653). Nursing researchers Dufault and Martocchio (1985) define hope as a "confident but uncertain expectation of achieving a future good which, to the hoping person, is realistically possible and personally significant" (p. 380). The philosopher Nunn (2005) argues that "if *A* hopes that *p*, then, *A* is uncertain whether *p* will happen, *A* believes that *p* is possible, *A* desires *p*, and, *A* judges *p* to be good in some respect" (p. 71; see also Day 1969). And, the philosopher Bovens (1999) defines hope as the conjunction of belief, desire and mentally imagining the sought-after outcome. These definitions identify key attributes of hope that are combined here into the following integrative definition: *hope is future-oriented belief, desire, and mental imagining surrounding a valued outcome that is uncertain but possible.*



A.J. Howell and D.J. Larsen, *Understanding Other-Oriented Hope*,
SpringerBriefs in Well-Being and Quality of Life Research,
DOI 10.1007/978-3-319-15007-9_3

Although these (single and integrated) definitions do not refer to hope held in the interest of others, neither do they preclude such a possibility. One can interpret the phrases *apply to one's own life, personally significant, good in some respect,* and *valued* as inclusive of events that people hope will transpire for significant others (i.e., in contrast with alternative phrasing which might have more directly referred to advancing only one's own interests). Indeed, Lazarus (1999) acknowledges the possibility of others being the target of one's hopes, and Nunn (2005) qualifies the final component of her analysis of hope with the phrase *morally good*—that is, taking into account the interests of others—in the case of viewing hope as a virtue. However, other-oriented hope can be made explicit by defining it in a manner that builds upon the earlier definitions of hope: we define other-oriented hope as *future-oriented belief, desire, and mental imagining surrounding a valued outcome of another person that is uncertain but possible.*

Hope is classified by Lazarus (1991, 1999) as an emotion; it reflects anticipated positive goal attainment and it generally involves an overall state of activation or readiness to engage in behaviour. Supporting the view of hope as an emotion, Averill et al. (1990) showed that hope shares several similarities with the emotions of love and anger, including that they are difficult to control, that they affect thinking and behaviour, and that they are shared, universal experiences. However, in reflecting upon the *problematic* status of hope as an emotion, Lazarus (1991, 1999) emphasizes that hope does not require a clear action tendency, does not have a readily identifiable underlying psychophysiology, and does not depend on the ability to influence the desired outcome. Lazarus (1991, 1999) also argues that hope could be viewed as "a cognitive (emotion-focused) coping process" (Lazarus 1991, p. 285) typically called upon under states of duress. As an emotion or a coping process, Lazarus (1991, 1999) emphasizes that hope can involve a blend of both positive and negative judgments and affects, because of the uncertainty of the occurrence of the hoped-for outcome, and that hope can be either approach- or avoidance-oriented. In addition to being construed as an emotion or as a coping process, hope has also been viewed variously as a cognition, disposition, state, and virtue (e.g., Lazarus 1999; Snyder 2002).

## 3.3 Differentiation of Hope from Related States

In keeping with Lazarus' (1991, 1999) view of hope as an emotion or an emotion-focused coping process, Roseman et al. (1990) compared hope with other emotional states. They had undergraduate students recall instances in which they experienced specific positive and negative emotions (e.g., hope, joy, fear, anger); students then made ratings concerning their appraisal of the situation (e.g., the predictability of the outcome, the extent to which they felt powerful or powerless in the situation). Results showed that hope was characterized by students as a discrete positive emotion which reflects the anticipation of attaining a *motive-consistent* outcome or avoiding a *motive-inconsistent outcome*, with such outcomes judged to have a relatively low certainty of occurrence. Hope was differentiable from other positive emotions; for example, in contrast to hope, joy was seen as involving greater certainty.

With an aim to elucidate features of hope in particular, Bruininks and Malle (2005) conducted folk analyses of the attributes of hope relative to several other states: optimism, joy, desire, wanting, and wishing. In their first study, undergraduate participants provided a description of these states. Overall, hope was viewed by young adults as a positive emotion surrounding the anticipation of a positive event, one function of which was to mobilize approach-related behaviour. Relative to optimism, descriptions of hope reflected greater importance, lower likelihood of attainment, and less personal control. Hope was also seen as being distinguishable from wish and desire, as the latter two involve low expectation of attainment and low personal control. Relative to the anticipation-related emotions (including hope), joy was seen as less future-oriented and less object- or event-oriented.

In a second study by Bruininks and Malle (2005), participants generated stories regarding the occurrence of hope and related states and then rated the degree of personal control they exerted over the situation, the importance of the outcome, and the likelihood of the outcome. Relative to the other states, stories regarding hope depicted such elements as a future orientation, low personal control, low ability to take action, and low likelihood of success. On the ratings subsequently made on the stories, hope was differentiable from optimism and joy in that hoped-for events were perceived as more important, less certain, and involving less personal control. Also, relative to desire and wanting, hope involved less control and greater importance. In a third study, multidimensional scaling was employed to differentiate hope from the remaining states, based on additional analysis of stories generated in the second study. Hope was differentiated from the other states in a two-dimensional space of personal control and subjective likelihood, with hope being characterized as low control and moderate likelihood, optimism involving moderate control and high likelihood, joy involving high control and high likelihood, wishing involving low control and low likelihood and, finally, desire/wanting involving high control and low likelihood.

Of relevance to the differentiation of hope and optimism demonstrated by Bruininks and Malle (2005), subsequent work has upheld the distinction: Bryant and Cvengros (2004) used structural equation modeling to demonstrate the differentiation of hope and optimism, ultimately concluding that hope was oriented toward goal-attainment whereas optimism concerned expectations about future outcomes more generally. Alarcon et al. (2013) used meta-analysis to show that the correlates of hope and optimism differed, with hope being more closely associated with stress and happiness, and optimism being more closely associated with personality variables such as self-esteem.

## 3.4 Conceptual Analyses of Hope

A number of hope theorists and researchers have offered conceptual analyses of the characteristics of hope. These analyses reveal the many dimensions along which hopes can vary. While these dimensions have largely been identified by analyses of self-oriented hope, reflecting the typical focus within hope studies, we argue later that these dimensions are likely to apply equally well to hope directed toward others.

On the basis of their empirical investigation into lay understandings of hope reviewed above, Averill et al. (1990) argue in support of four *rules of hope*: Hope should involve a realistic appraisal of probability, hope should concern objects that are personally or socially acceptable (i.e., reflecting values, mores, or ethical virtues), hope should concern outcomes deemed important, and hope should provoke action [Averill et al. noted that an exception to this latter rule is that of other-oriented hope, which is often under limited personal influence; see also Day (1969)].

In their conceptual analysis of hope from a nursing perspective, Benzein and Saveman (1998) identify the following major elements of hope: future orientation, positive expectation, intentionality, activity, realism, goal setting, and interconnectedness. Notably, in expanding upon the latter element, the authors identified that "hope could include the self and/or others" (p. 325). Dufault and Martocchio (1985), based upon their work with terminally ill persons, identify six dimensions of hope: affective (including predominantly positive feelings but also feelings related to uncertainty), cognitive (including judgments of the possibility of various hope objects), behavioural (including direct action toward attainment of hope objects), affiliative (including the individual's relationships with other people, other living things, and/or higher beings), temporal (including a future-orientation) and contextual (including the patient's recent experience of loss or stress). Importantly, they describe the affective dimension as including outcomes that are desirable *for another person* and they describe the affiliative dimension as including *concern for others*. These latter attributes are congruent with the existence of vicarious hope.

Morse and Doberneck (1995), based on their analysis of patients undergoing heart transplant, patients with spinal-cord injury, breast cancer patients, and mothers intending to continue breastfeeding upon return to work, identify seven *universal and abstract* components of hope: realistically appraising the threat; envisioning of alternative possibilities and goal-setting; bracing for negative outcomes; realistically appraising personal and external resources; soliciting support from others; ongoing evaluation of the goal and the means to achieve it; and the "determination to endure" (p. 278), or resiliency. Also in a nursing context, Stephenson (1991) identifies key attributes of hope as including a meaningful object; the simultaneous involvement of thoughts, feelings, behaviours, and relationships; anticipation; and positive future orientation.

The dimensions emphasized by Novotny (1989) within an illness context are that hope: is future-oriented; involves active engagement; is an inner resource; reflects possibility; is relational; and concerns issues of importance. Also within a healthcare context, Simpson (2004) identifies four key elements of hope: the role of desires/wants; a connection with values/goals; the role of imagination and uncertainty; and the action aspect of hope. Hendricks-Ferguson (1997) argues that critical attributes of hope among adolescents with cancer include positive thinking, realistic future-oriented goals, a positive support system, and a positive future for self *or others*. Finally, Haase et al. (1992), in a conceptual analysis contrasting hope, spirituality, acceptance, and self-transcendence from a nursing perspective, characterizes hope as future-oriented, action-oriented, goal-oriented, and as involving uncertainty.

Schrank et al. (2010) factor analyzed 60-items taken from three existing hope scales. Four dimensions of hope arose, labelled *trust and confidence* (e.g., goal striving, positive past experience), *positive future orientation* (e.g., looking forward, making plans), *social relations and personal value* (e.g., feeling loved and needed), and *lack of perspective* (e.g., feeling trapped, becoming uninvolved).

Pettit (2004) emphasizes that hope is characterized by a desire for an outcome that is uncertain but possible and a personal resolve to act in congruence with the outcome. Pettit further argues that, defined in this way, hope is both rational and ubiquitous. McGeer (2004) argues that hope involves "taking an agential interest in the future" (p. 104). Both Pettit and McGeer stipulate that even in the case that one is not able to directly impact the desired outcome, the presence of hope instills a more general fortitude to persevere, to engage, and to live. Webb (2007), on this note, distinguishes between hope that is open-ended and that which is goal-oriented. Tennen et al. (2002) emphasize that trust is a significant aspect of hope, and specified that trust occurs at the confluence of low certainty, low control, and (despite the first two qualities) positive anticipation. Scioli and colleagues label the key dimensions of hope as mastery, attachment, survival, and spiritual (Scioli et al. 2011, p. 79). Hope, from this view, involves personal and shared strivings energized by both approach (e.g., mastery) and avoidance (e.g., safety) motivations and occurring within a supportive interpersonal and faith-based context.

In the most influential psychological perspective on hope, and one previously described in Chap. 1, Snyder and colleagues posit that hope is "a positive motivational state that is based on an interactively derived sense of successful (a) agency (goal-directed energy), and (b) pathways (planning to meet goals)" (Snyder et al. 1991, p. 287). According to this view, hope-agency beliefs provide motivation to pursue valued goals, and hope-pathways beliefs provide plausible routes to meet those goals. This conceptualization emphasizes the cognitive component of hope, but it also acknowledges an important role of positive emotions (especially upon goal achievement) and experiences of vitality during goal pursuit (Snyder 2002).

**Box 3.1: Hope Theories and Individual Differences**

For the past decade, I (D. L.) have taught a senior university level course on hope, entitled *Hope and the Helping Relationship*. In the course we address many different theories of hope including multidimensional approaches such as that of Dufault and Martocchio (1985) and, of course, Snyder's (2002) cognitive-behavioural goals-focused approach. While differences in hope theories are often disconcerting to students early in the course, I have seen a trend in how these theories are taken up by various students. Attempting to provide a balanced introduction to hope theories, we systematically review the theories identifying both our appreciation and constructive critique. For one of the assignments in the course, students outline and discuss the theories which align or converge with their own personal understandings of hope. It has been interesting to note that, predictably, about a quarter of the class will be taken with Snyder's cognitive-behavioural orientation to hope, particularly drawn to the self-oriented focus on goals, while the remainder of the class will be drawn to more multidimensional understandings of hope.

In sum, hope is most often construed as an emotion or as an emotion-based coping process. Hope is differentiable from other, related states such as optimism, joy, and desire. Hope has various key defining characteristics which include uncertainty, limited controllability, realism, positive anticipation of the attainment of desired outcomes or the avoidance of undesired outcomes, goal-setting and planning, a general motivational energy, future orientation, high perceived importance, and contexts of challenge or loss. Other-oriented hope was, on numerous occasions, referenced by researchers and theorists in their discussion of the attributes of general hope. Moreover, it is likely that other-oriented hope has similar characteristics to self-oriented hope; that is, other-oriented hope will involve the positive anticipation that others deemed important to us will meet desired outcomes or avoid undesired outcomes in the future, despite the uncertainty of those outcomes, the (possibly) negative plight of the other, and low levels of control over producing those outcomes. Therefore, other-oriented hope will tend to resemble self-oriented hope. Although the target of the hoped for event is someone other than the self, the experience of other-oriented hope will, by and large, appear similar to that of self-oriented hope.

Given this account of the definition, elements, and dimensions of other-oriented hope we can, in the next chapter, examine evidence for its existence.

**Box 3.2: An Application of Hope and Other-Oriented Hope**
The field of education has taken up hope as a vital factor in learning. Both social justice concerns (e.g., te Riele 2010) along with more individualistic (Snyder 2002) orientations to hope appear in the research on teaching. Hope practices in schools are often tied to the curriculum in innovative ways that reflect a focus on both self- and other-oriented hope. Some of the most fascinating hope work appears in the classroom practices of teachers who both lead with hope and respond to their students' interests in hope. One such teacher, Ms. Bonn, developed a writing reflection unit on hope for her grade 11 and 12 High School special needs students. Integrated into their Career

and Life Management program, the students were given a special blank journal, called their *Hope Journal*. Over a series of eight lessons, each week the teacher presented a new topic on hope as a springboard for class discussion followed by time for individual journaling. The first topic invited students to consider what hope was as it applied to themselves, and perhaps more importantly, what filled them with hope. The teacher shared her own story of a past camping trip and the hopeful feeling she had as she recounted that experience. Students were invited to follow similarly. The experience triggered strong emotional memories and thoughts about hope.

With respect to other-oriented hope, the second lesson offers particular insight. Rather than directing students to focus on themselves, Ms. Bonn 'primed' her students. She asked them to consider the hopes they held for others. Recognizing that sharing hope can invite personal vulnerability (Simpson 2004), she felt that an other-oriented focus on hope would be less intimidating and may also be easier for students who sometimes struggle with self-reflection. Ms. Bonn began her lesson with her own story of hopes for her father. Her sharing spurred a powerful class dialogue as students took risks to share their own hopes for loved ones, deeply meaningful hopes including hopes for mental health and addictions recovery, renewed health for ill loved ones, and an end to abusive relationships they witnessed in others. The students hoped that loved ones would find peace, hope, and happiness. Aware that they had little power to implement the hopes they held for others, the class discussed how they might share their hope with others, conveying that they loved, cared for, and believed in the possibility of a good future for those they loved. Following this class discussion, Ms. Bonn found that she needed to provide extra writing time for students because the students had much to say. She was particularly taken with the impact of this writing session on the class as she felt that the students had come to a better understanding of each other and that the group discussion had created a more cohesive and empathetic classroom environment.

## References

Alarcon, G. M., Bowling, N. A., & Khazon, S. (2013). Great expectations: A meta-analytic examination of optimism and hope. *Personality and Individual Differences, 54*, 821–827.

Averill, J. R., Catlin, G., & Chon, K. K. (1990). *Rules of hope*. New York: Springer.

Benzein, E., & Saveman, B. I. (1998). Nurses' perception of hope in patients with cancer: A palliative care perspective. *Cancer Nursing, 21*, 10–16.

Bovens, L. (1999). The value of hope. *Philosophy and Phenomenological Research, 59*, 667–681.

Bruininks, P., & Malle, B. F. (2005). Distinguishing hope from optimism and related affective states. *Motivation and Emotion, 29*, 327–355.

Bryant, F. B., & Cvengros, J. A. (2004). Distinguishing hope and optimism: Two sides of a coin, or two separate coins? *Journal of Social and Clinical Psychology, 23*, 273–302.

Day, J. P. (1969). Hope. *American Philosophical Quarterly, 6*, 89–102.

Dufault, K., & Martocchio, B. C. (1985). Hope: Its spheres and dimensions. *Nursing Clinics of North America, 20*, 379–391.

Haase, J. E., Britt, T., Coward, D. D., Kline Leidy, N., & Penn, P. E. (1992). Simultaneous concept analysis of spiritual perspective, hope, acceptance and self-transcendence. *Journal of Nursing Scholarship, 24*, 141–147.

Hendricks-Ferguson, V. (1997). An analysis of the concept of hope in the adolescent cancer patient. *Journal of Pediatric Oncology Nursing, 14*, 73–80.

Lazarus, R. S. (1991). *Emotion and adaptation*. New York: Oxford University Press.

Lazarus, R. S. (1999). Hope: An emotion and a vital coping resource against despair. *Social Research, 66*, 653–678.

McGeer, V. (2004). The art of good hope. *Annals of the American Academy of Political and Social Science, 592*, 100–127.

Morse, J. M., & Doberneck, B. (1995). Delineating the concept of hope. *Journal of Nursing Scholarship, 27*, 277–285.

Novotny, M. L. (1989). Assessment of hope in patients with cancer: Development of an instrument. *Oncology Nursing Forum, 16*, 57–61.

Nunn, B. V. (2005). Getting clear what hope is. In J. A. Eliott (Ed.), *Interdisciplinary perspectives on hope* (pp. 63–77). New York: Nova Science Publishers.

Pettit, P. (2004). Hope and its place in mind. *Annals of the American Academy of Political and Social Science, 592*, 152–165.

Roseman, I. J., Spindel, M. S., & Jose, P. E. (1990). Appraisals of emotion-eliciting events: Testing a theory of discrete emotions. *Journal of Personality and Social Psychology, 59*, 899–915.

Schrank, B., Mag, A. W., Sibitz, I., & Lauber, C. (2010). Development and validation of an integrative scale to assess hope. *Health Expectations, 14*, 417–428.

Scioli, A., Ricci, M., Nyugen, T., & Scioli, R. (2011). Hope: Its nature and measurement. *Psychology of Religion and Spirituality, 3*, 78–97.

Simpson, C. (2004). When hope makes us vulnerable: A discussion of patient-healthcare provider interactions in the context of hope. *Bioethics, 18*, 428–447.

Snyder, C. R. (2002). Hope theory: Rainbows in the mind. *Psychological Inquiry, 13*, 1047–1084.

Snyder, C. R., Irving, L., & Anderson, J. R. (1991). Hope and health: measuring the will and the ways. In C. R. Snyder & D. R. Forsyth (Eds.), *Handbook of social and clinical psychology: The health perspective* (pp. 285–305). Elmsford, New York: Pergamon Press.

Stephenson, C. (1991). The concept of hope revisited for nursing. *Journal of Advanced Nursing, 16*, 1456–1461.

Te Riele, K. (2010). Philosophy of hope: Concepts and applications for working with marginalised youth. *Journal of Youth Studies, 13*, 35–46.

Tennen, H., Affleck, G., & Tennen, R. (2002). Clipped feathers: The theory and measurement of hope. *Psychological Inquiry, 13*, 311–317.

Webb, D. (2007). Modes of hoping. *History of the Human Sciences, 20*, 65–83.

# Chapter 4
# Research Yielding Evidence of Other-Oriented Hope

## 4.1 General

*Every teacher and parent knows how to hope for another's benefit, even at his or her own expense. Sacrifices of time, wealth, and psychic energy are made in the hope of another's future well-being. Hope for another's benefit excludes some hopes for one's own, because not both are possible.*
—Godfrey 1987, p. 136

To date, research on other-oriented hope has largely been descriptive in nature, reflecting its relatively nascent status within hope studies. Descriptive research has as its goal the observation and documentation of a phenomenon and its characteristics. The majority of quantitative research on other-oriented hope has sought to link the holding of vicarious hope with other outcomes of interest, such as associating the presence of other-oriented hope with well-being or adaptive coping. In addition to correlational research, quantitative approaches have, on rare occasions, employed experimental and quasi-experimental approaches (e.g., tracking changes in hope following an intervention or other experimental manipulation). Quantitative research has, at times, involved direct requests to participants to identify outcomes for which they are hopeful, later categorizing the reported hopes as self- or other-oriented, thereby allowing for the quantification of different forms of hope and for examination of associations between other-oriented hope and other attributes of hope such as their importance or their probability.

Qualitative research in this area most often makes use of semi-structured interviews regarding vulnerable individuals' hope, such as the hope of patients or of elderly individuals. In this form of research, interview questions are typically open-ended (e.g., *What is it that you hope for?*), in which case the verbalized or written responses are subsequently content analyzed (Thorne 2008) and hope themes or categories (including those related to other-oriented hope) are induced. Conversely, interview questions can be more narrowly focused upon the possibility of others being the target of one's hope (e.g., *What hope do you hold for your child?*). Qualitative researchers also employ content analysis of journal entries or other



A.J. Howell and D.J. Larsen, *Understanding Other-Oriented Hope*,
SpringerBriefs in Well-Being and Quality of Life Research,
DOI 10.1007/978-3-319-15007-9_4

materials (e.g., psychotherapy session content) to yield evidence concerning hope and vicarious hope. Some researchers have interviewed participants on more than one occasion, adding a longitudinal component to the research design and allowing for the detection of changes in hope content over time. Finally, a number of syntheses of qualitative research have examined large bodies of studies simultaneously, yielding evidence as to whether other-oriented hope emerges as a consistent theme or content category across studies.

Other-oriented hope is likely to reveal itself in some domains of everyday life more than others. Specifically, other-oriented hope should be most prominent within situations that either sensitize people toward the vulnerability of others or that reduce people's preoccupation with, or judgment of the relative importance of, their own circumstances. These domains are reflected in research which has examined or uncovered instances of vicarious hope: hope among parents of ill children, hope among informal caregivers, hope among formal caregivers, hope among those with serious illnesses, and hope among teachers. Note that research reviewed within these domains is limited to that which explicitly examined other-oriented hope, not hope in general. For example, although research has supported an association between parental (self-oriented) hope and coping with a child's illness (e.g., Kirpalani et al. 2000), only research concerning parental other-oriented hope is included in the section that follows. Finally, we also review research that has examined the more general occurrence of other-oriented hope.

## 4.2 Other-Oriented Hope Among Parents of Ill Children

It is likely that parents hold hope for their healthy children, including hope regarding their children's health, their well-being, and their future accomplishments. However, the study of parental hope toward children has especially concerned children experiencing significant illnesses. Wong and Heriot (2007) define *vicarious hope* as hope held for another's future, and identify its occurrence in the context of parental hope for their ill children. They showed, among a sample of parents of children with autism and related conditions, that other-oriented hope toward their children (measured with such items as *I generally believe that my child's future will be very active*) was positively correlated with parental personal hope. In a subsequent study, Wong and Heriot (2008) showed that, among a sample of parents of children with cystic fibrosis, other-oriented hope was associated with lower parental depression and anxiety. Most recently, Faso et al. (2013) showed that, among mothers and fathers of children with autism spectrum disorder, other-oriented hope was modestly and non-significantly related to agency and pathways thinking of parents, but was significantly related to parental life satisfaction, low parental depression, and low parental stress.

Larson (1998) conducted in-depth case studies of six mothers of children aged 5–11 who had significant disabilities, based upon extensive interviews and direct observation. A key theme uncovered in qualitative analysis of the findings was the mothers' grappling with a paradox: "...understanding the impaired condition of their child and yet fully embracing a more hopeful future as well as guarding against a painful one" (p. 871). A direct quotation from one of the participants illustrates this challenge:

> Well, the difficult thing is that you always want your child to be normal, to be [...] your dream is you know, to see them running around and maybe be normal. That's the difficult part, because you know in your heart that you can't, that you're never gonna see that. I don't know [...] I know she'll probably walk. I don't know when, but I know. I know that is my dream to see her walk. But I know she is not going to be able to see, she's always gonna be blind. But she, even though she walks, she's not going to be a normal one, one of them. (p. 868)

In a study of 546 parents of children with Down syndrome, Truitt et al. (2012) measured the degree of parental agency and pathways thinking concerning goals they held for their children in six domains (social skills, behaviour, education, independence, mental health, physical health, and *other*). Findings revealed that the degree of pathways thinking across these domains, but not the degree of agency thinking, positively predicted the degree of parental adaptation to their child's challenges. Therefore, other-oriented hope among parents was associated with resilience in the form of solution-oriented planning in the face of their child's illness-related vulnerability.

Stein et al. (2007) asked 29 parents of adolescents with mental disorders (primarily schizophrenia or bipolar disorder) to list up to 10 things that they *hoped would happen for their adult child.* Hope statements were classified into the following categories, ordered from most to least common in terms of percentage of parental hope: personal relationships (22.4 %), independence (17.4 %), employment (15.9 %), being happy or living fully (12.2 %), education (11.6 %), mental health issues (10.8 %), self-improvement (5.0 %), and religion/spiritual (0.7 %). Therefore, when explicitly asked to consider their hope toward their vulnerable children, parents generated many examples of other-oriented hope, emphasizing aspects of their child's future which would reflect on their overall well-being and adaptive functioning.

Evidence of parental hope toward critically ill newborns was presented by Amendolia (2010). For example, in the case of a girl who was born three months premature with severe respiratory distress, Amendolia states:

> Watching her progress slowly with the feedings and weight gain has been difficult, but both parents remain optimistic and believe that their baby will be coming home by the time her due date arrives. They set goals for her weight gain and believe that she can achieve them. (p. 142)

Kylma and Juvakka (2007) interviewed nine parents of adolescents with cancer. Parents were interviewed on three occasions, during which "they were asked to describe their hope during their child's course of illness and the factors associated with their hope" (p. 264). They identified other-oriented hope in the form of positive wishes of parents regarding their child's outcomes: "I wish that the life would be good for my daughter"; "Hope for the normal life"; and "Of course I hope that my daughter will have her faith in God also in the future" (p. 265).

Other-oriented hope also emerged in a qualitative study of 19 parents of children with developmental disabilities (Kausar et al. 2003). Parents were interviewed in a semi-structured fashion with such questions as, *Regarding your experience as a parent of a child with disability, what does hope mean to you?*, and *Can you think of any events that have either enhanced or diminished your feelings of hope?* Eight themes emerged as common across the sample, labelled care and compassion, realistic understanding, focus on abilities, transformation, unified family, spiritual beliefs, social support, and professionals' attitudes. The researchers provided examples of instances of other-oriented hope emerging within the *realistic understanding* theme ("So my only hope is as long as he lives…he lives a comfortable life…then I am satisfied"; p. 39) and within the *focus on abilities* theme ("…that she can live an independent life with some support"; p. 40).

Cohn et al. (2000) argue that a family-centred provision of services by occupational therapists must take into account parental hope for their child's future. They conducted semi-structured interviews with eight parents of five children who exhibited sensory modulation disorders. Interviews included the question, *What are your expectations and/or hopes for therapy?* Answers were content-analyzed and categorized, yielding three child-focused outcomes of social participation, self-regulation, and perceived competence and two parent-focused outcomes of learning strategies to support the child and personal validation. An example of a child-focused hope (falling within the perceived competence category) was a parent's comment that, "What I want for Harry is, like, happiness or contentment or satisfaction with himself…it is bigger than just self-confidence but includes self-confidence…I wish he could get pleasure from what he himself can do and who he is as a person" (p. 39). An example of a parent-focused hope (falling within the personal validation category) was a parent's comment that, "I want confirmation that I'm not 'weird', that Harry isn't 'bad', that there are other children like Harry, that his problems are 'real' and not just in my head. I want to be accepted and bolstered for what I do for Harry rather than people thinking that I'm a bad mother" (p. 40). Parent-focused and child-focused hopes reveal the necessary coexistence in parents of ill children of both self- and other-interest.

## 4.3 Other-Oriented Hope Among Informal Caregivers

Outside of the role of parenting a child, it has been emphasized that caring for another person often involves hoping for their future well-being. Other-oriented hope is an important component to supporting a family member in their recovery from schizophrenia (Bamforth and Pederson 2008). Tibaldi and Govers (2012) note that:

> The *reasonable hope* of recovery also represents an indispensable shared objective, which is often missing, to be embraced by all those people affected by a psychotic episode, their families, and health professionals to promote their effective interaction toward a common horizon. (p. 113)

Bland and Darlington (2002) interviewed 16 family members of people with primarily schizophrenia or bipolar disorder about hope in relation to mental illness. Other-oriented hope included longing for a loved one's recovery (e.g., "…so all through her illness we'd continue to hope that she would get better and hope that, you know, there'd be a cure for schizophrenia…"; p. 63). Other examples of hope among family members were more self-oriented or were mixed in their orientation, such as hoping for personal strength in order to continue to help the ill family member. Overall, the researchers conclude that vicarious hope among family members emerged among a majority of the families interviewed.

Hernandez et al. (2013) also studied family members' hope toward loved ones with schizophrenia. Family members of 54 Latino persons with schizophrenia completed a semi-structured measure of family burden and the Hope for the Patient's Future Scale (Kopelowicz et al. 2003). The latter measure consisted of 20 items on which the family member rated their level of hope, including *the illness of your family member gets better* and *your family member will be able to develop his/her own goals for the future* (p. 701). Results showed that a higher degree of hope toward the ill family member was associated with lower family burden, even after controlling for the length of patients' illnesses.

In related research, Kopelowicz et al. (2003) measured hope (with the Hope for Patient's Future Scale) and family burden among family members of 92 patients diagnosed with schizophrenia spectrum disorders. Patients were then randomly assigned to a skills training condition (emphasizing medication adherence and symptom management) or treatment-as-usual condition. Patient groups met four times per week whereas family member groups met once weekly. No differences emerged across conditions on the levels of family member hope or burden at the end of the 3-month treatment period or at a six-month follow-up. The researchers reported that levels of hope were high and levels of burden were low throughout the study period. While this study failed to show elevations in other-oriented hope as a function of specific treatment provided to the ill family member, it did demonstrate that hope directed toward the ill individual can be high among family members of those with schizophrenia, and that this tends to be accompanied by reduced experience of burden.

In a study by Friedman-Yakoobian et al. (2009), 51 adult relatives of individuals with schizophrenia and related conditions rated their other-oriented hope in response to the question, *In general, how hopeful are you concerning your relative's future?*; they also completed measures of burden, psychological distress, and past-month coping behaviours. Higher hope was associated with lesser burden, distress, and maladaptive coping (especially behavioural disengagement), but was unrelated to illness characteristics.

In a review of studies concerning hope and schizophrenia, Kylma et al. (2006) identified hope of caregivers toward the future well-being of the person with schizophrenia as a significant theme. Karanci (1995), for example, showed that about 54 % of family caregivers held hope that their relative will become well in the future.

Turning to a focus upon physical disorders, Holtslander et al. (2005) interviewed 10 informal caregivers of family members with terminal illnesses. The interview began with the prompt, *Tell me about hope*. Coding of open-ended responses to this question revealed that caregiver hope was aimed toward the patient, the caregivers themselves, and the caregivers' families. Examples of other-oriented hope provided by respondents included: "We're hoping she gets through this with the least amount of pain and the most dignity she can", and "I hope she stays healthy" (p. 287). Similarly, Patel (1996) interviewed 20 spouses of critically ill adults. In response to the open-ended question, *What are you hoping for?*, 18 of the spouses verbalized instances of vicarious hope, such as hoping that the patient's life would return to normal, hoping that the patient would live a long life, and hoping that the patient would adjust to lifestyle changes and experience little suffering.

Duggleby et al. (2011) identified examples of other-oriented hope among the directed written journal entries of 10 family caregivers of those with cancer. Qualitative examples of other-oriented hope emerging in the study included, "Hope? Maybe it will be a better day tomorrow for her – there ought to be some good or better days for her yet" (p. 465). Holtslander and Duggleby (2009) conducted interviews with 13 women aged 60 years and older who had cared for their spouses with terminal cancer (the spouses had died within the past year). Interviews included questions such as *What thoughts do you have about hope? and What does hope mean for you right now?* The researchers identified that their participants' hope concerned themselves, their future, or their family. Moreover, they argued that *finding new meaning and purpose* was an important aspect of the search for new hope, and they identified specific instances of other-oriented hope falling within this domain: "I think any hope that I have for the future will be in watching my grandchildren grow and mature, taking part in their lives and being there for all of them if they need me" (p. 396); and "Hope for the future, yeah, because I've got children and I've got grandchildren" (p. 396).

Duggleby et al. (2009) identified examples of other-oriented hope among answers to open-ended interview questions posed to 17 caregivers of family members living with Alzheimer's Disease, including "…I'm hoping that he can be at least the way he is from one day to another" (p. 518). However, it was also noted that caregivers held more hope for themselves than for their loved ones, perhaps reflecting the nature of their loved one's ailments and the burden experienced by caregivers in this context (e.g., "I'm hoping I can manage with him…", p. 518).

In a study of persons with dementia living in long-term care, Duggleby et al. (2013) interviewed 13 family caregivers. Participants kept a hope journal, and underwent a semi-structured interview regarding their hope (e.g., *Tell me about hope*). Journal entries and interview responses were thematically interpreted, with an overall theme of *hope and connection* emerging. Several examples of other-oriented hope were identified by the researchers: "every day…she'll be alert and responsive…and I guess hope is that she will stay like that for a long time" (p. 5); "When I think of the word HOPE in relation to Dad, I know he didn't want to end up with his memory failing and being dependent on others for his care. So my hope is he will pass peacefully in his sleep without losing total dignity" (p. 5); "So you hope that you can somehow give them some happiness" (p. 5). Other hope identified by family caregivers was more clearly self-oriented hope: "In my life? Hope for a long, peaceful, and healthy life…and- and not ending up in the same way…" (p. 5); "It is certainly my fervent hope that something takes me quickly and painlessly before I become demented" (p. 6).

Gebhardt et al. (2011) interviewed family members of 21 patients between 15 and 21 years old who had recently suffered an acquired brain injury. One of the semi-structured interview questions asked directly about hope for the patient's future. The researchers report that all caregivers were able to identify hope related to their loved one, and hope typically centred on the patient returning to school or work and otherwise resuming their previous lives. As an example, one mother in the study stated, "I hope that she'll be as close to the [person] that we had before the accident as possible…Hoping that she will be well enough to go back at school… I hope she'll be as much on her own as she can possibly be" (p. 7).

A related study involved 22 family members of 16 coma patients in intensive care (Verhaeghe et al. 2007). The family members underwent two semi-structured interviews concerning their experiences, the first soon after the patient's admission to hospital and the second upon the patient regaining consciousness or upon the patient's death. Results suggested that hope involved a *stepped* process, wherein the nature of family member hope changed over the course of time. Initially, family member hope was directed toward the injuries being slight or the loved one still being alive. Upon seeing the patient, survival of the loved one became a major focus of family member hope, as in these examples: "Well, he's lying there in a coma. You can see that it's bad, the machines, the tubes, there's a reason why they're there. And they tell you it's not good, he's hanging by a thread, we can hope that he survives, but you can't hope for anything more than that" (p. 734); "And then comes the moment of truth. I will never forget it. All the hopes you had explode right in your face. You see him and you know, all you can hope for is that he survives" (p. 736). In the case of a lack of progress by the patient, family member hope was described as directed toward their loved ones not suffering or knowing their family is at their side. In the case of the patient's death, family members held hope that the loved one's death has meaning; for example, in relation to organ donation.

A man's hope concerning his partner's AIDS-related dementia was studied by Kelly (2007). In this case, when hope for a cure disappeared, other-oriented hope took the form of hoping for the patient's death. As stated by Kelly, "As treatments kept Tom alive yet did not restore him to his former self, Matthew no longer knew where to find hope. He could only hope that an end would come, and soon" (p. 872).

Another study in this domain focused upon 11 men whose wives had breast cancer (Duggleby et al. 2012a). The men underwent two semi-structured telephone interviews, which included questions such as *What gives you hope*? and *Tell me about hope*. Thematic analysis of responses to such questions yielded an overall theme identified as *engaging hope*, and subthemes of finding balance, discovering what works, and focusing on the positive. With regard to the overarching theme, the researchers identified that hope was both self-oriented and other-oriented. One patient stated, "I have hope for her and for my family … hoping that something good would happen" (p. 403).

There is some evidence that other-oriented hope can develop as a result of supporting the family members of an ill loved-one. In a quasi-experiment by Redlich et al. (2010), the hopes of 97 family members of those with a mental illness were assessed before and after they participated in either a 45 h didactic intervention aimed at enhancing communication and cooperation within the family or a control condition consisting of a social gathering for families. Snyder's Adult Hope Scale was used to assess family member's own hope, and a modified version of the scale was used to assess family members' hope toward their ill loved one. Results showed that self-oriented hope did not change from pre- to post-assessment for either group. However, the experimental group showed a greater enhancement of hope toward the family member after the intervention relative to before the intervention, whereas no such change occurred in the control group.

In a recent synthesis of the literature concerning hope among informal caregivers, Duggleby et al. (2010) reviewed 14 qualitative studies. Their analysis identified three categories of hope, labeled old/lost hope and new hope, short-term specific hope, and long-term specific hope. The latter two types of hope were both identified as including other-oriented hope, such as short-term hope that a family member's health would improve, or that the family member would experience reduced suffering.

## 4.4 Other-Oriented Hope Among Formal Caregivers

Formal caregivers, such as psychotherapists, nurses, and physicians, harbour hopes for their clients as part of their role as care providers, with a lack of hope associated with burnout and compassion fatigue (e.g., Austin et al. 2013). In the psychotherapy context, the importance of therapist hope toward their clients was identified almost half a century ago by Frank (1968), and continues to be viewed as an important element of the therapeutic change process (e.g., Dufrane and Leclair 1984; Snyder et al. 1999). Despite the importance of therapist hope being identified by luminary psychotherapists such as Karen Horney (Manrique 1984), surprisingly little research directly concerns therapist hope for clients.

Coppock et al. (2010) conducted a naturalistic field study to examine client hope, therapist hope, and client improvement among 43 psychotherapy clients and 10 psychologists and counsellors. Using Snyder's State Hope Scale to measure hope within clients themselves and (in a modified version) hope held by therapists for their clients, results showed that therapist hope toward their clients was predictive of client progress. Interestingly, client hope was not related to client outcomes in this study.

Five counsellors working with women on probation or parole were interviewed regarding their views toward the role of hope for themselves and their clients and regarding work-related experiences that bolstered or reduced their hope (Flesaker and Larsen 2010). Qualitative interpretation of interview responses identified an overall theme of *maintaining a hope-seeking orientation*, and subthemes of *understandings of hope, life is a journey, hope maintained through life perspective, hope maintained by "down-to-earth" expectations,* and *finding hope is a learnable skill*. Within these subthemes, counsellors identified clients' hope concerning their own futures, counsellors' hope concerning themselves as counsellors, and counsellors' hope concerning their clients' futures. Counsellors' hope toward their clients emerged within the theme of *understandings of hope*, where specific examples provided by the counsellor respondents included: "Hope is when we see possibilities, when we see potential in ourselves, when we see potential in others, when there's a greater good" (p. 68); "[Hope means] that I or anyone else can become who [we were] created to be" (p. 68); "I've said 'believe' a lot and I think belief and hope for me, kind of, coincide. If you believe in someone, you have hope, right?" (p. 69); and "I have hope when, even if a woman is out of [the correctional facility] for a period of time and she ends up going back. I have hope that next time she journeys out that she's found some skills ... that that piece of that journey is only going to make her stronger for next time" (p. 71).

Larsen et al. (2013) conducted an in-depth investigation of psychologists' hope in relation to their clients, including the importance of the therapist conveying "a genuine belief in, and hope for, the client" (p. 3). Five psychologists working with 11 clients underwent interviews, during which videotape play-back of a recent psychotherapy session was used to encourage psychologists' reflection on the role of their own hope within the session. Qualitative analysis of interview content suggested three core themes: psychologist self-influence on hope (including self-dialogue concerning imagined future work with the client); client factors impacting psychologist hope (including the presence of client progress); and psychologist hope within the therapeutic relationship (including the idea of *empathic hoping*, wherein psychologists' hope for the client reflects the client's own hope). Larsen et al. further note that the psychologists' hope toward their clients was both outcome-oriented (i.e., hoping for alleviation of the client's presenting problem) and process-oriented (e.g., hoping for a strong working alliance with the client). This distinction between process- and outcome-oriented hope is unique within the literature on other-oriented hope. Counselling psychologists' hope toward their clients, and the significant role that it plays within the counselling process, was also evidenced in an analysis of two counselling cases surrounding the concept of unrealistic hope (Larsen et al. 2014).

Darlington and Bland (1999) interviewed six mental health professionals with the aim of revealing how they foster and maintain hope with clients experiencing serious mental illness. The following therapist observation was used to exemplify the role of therapist hope toward their client in fostering client hope and client progress:

> I think having a sense of hope is really, really important and that doesn't mean I suppose that, you know, they are going to be completely cured of mental illness. There's degrees of

> it, of hope, but I think you can certainly have a sense that your clients are going to be more functional in their lives and just basically have a little bit more control and a sense of happiness I guess. If you are not able to convey that to your clients I really don't think you should be working here. (p. 20)

Weingarten's (2010) construct of *reasonable hope*, defined as action-oriented hope toward achievable ends, is discussed in the context of family therapy. Rather than therapists *instilling* hope or *inspiring* hope, Weingarten suggests a "metaphor of accompaniment" (p. 11) in which hopes are co-created. One basis for such co-created hope is hope held by the therapist for the client, as in the example of a therapist struggling to adopt a reasonable hope for a client in a challenging situation involving imprisonment and the potential loss of custody over her children. Also in the context of family therapy, Flaskas (2007) speaks of the importance of the balance within the therapist of hope versus hopelessness concerning their clients' futures in order to respect both the possibility of change and the reality of the some families' situations. Flaskas also argues for a role for family therapy in exploring the importance of family members holding hope for each other when the individual is unable to hold such hope. Koenig and Spano (2007) speak of the general importance of social workers' hope for their clients' ability to grow and change, and the cultivation of such hope in social work education.

In the medical context, Wildes (1999), Pellegrino and Thomasma (1996), and Eliott and Olver (2002) identify that medical staff, perhaps by necessity, hold hope that treatment of their patients will be successful. Jevne (1991) encourages professional caregivers to ask themselves, among other questions, "What hope(s) do I have for this person?" (p. 171). Gadgeel (2011) discusses hope held by physicians toward their patients, posing the question: "How can I, as an oncologist, balance the hope that the next treatment I offer to my patients with advanced lung cancer will be effective with the realistic probability that benefit is unlikely?" (p. 2292; see Chap. 7 for a discussion of so-called *unrealistic* hope). However, Richardson et al. (2012) provide the following example of the dissociation between the provision of medical care and other-oriented hope (while nonetheless underscoring the potentially important role of other-oriented hope among informal caregivers of the patient): "Hoping is about anticipation and wanting things to go well. I leave hope up to the families and friends. I don't get into hoping at all. I don't consider myself to be a hoper but a fixer" (p. 688).

Gebhardt et al. (2011) conducted semi-structured interviews with nurses of 21 in-patients recently admitted following an acquired brain injury. The interview included the specific prompt to describe their hope for the patient's future. The researchers reported that nurses' hope often surrounded specific markers of patient progress in daily living, as in the following example: "I hope he'll be able to recover to a level where he can do things for himself as far as like going to the bathroom, being able to feed himself" (p. 8). In discussing the role of the healthcare providers' hope for their patients, Simpson (2004) considers the importance of the co-creation of patients' hope: "…being able to imagine with patients a variety of – potentially achievable, sustainable, or acceptable – 'futures' for themselves would be one way of enabling patients to discover hope" (p. 439).

## 4.5 Other-Oriented Hope Among Those with Serious Illnesses

There is evidence that other-oriented hope occurs frequently among those coping with life-threatening illnesses. Based upon interviews with 28 persons in the final phases of terminal cancer, including the question *What are you hoping for?*, Eliott and Olver (2009) identify instances of other-oriented hope, such as in the following example of avoidance-oriented vicarious hope: "I hope there won't be anything left that has to be a burden for my family. I just hope that when I've gone that there's nothing that is going to be left for other people to clean up" (p. 628). Another patient's hope was "that when my time comes that it's not too hard on the family. I don't want that" (p. 622). Eliott and Olver (2009) speculate that such hope is conducive to well-being because of the strengthening of relationships that occurs via other-oriented hope.

In an earlier paper, Eliott and Olver (2007) give the following example of a terminally ill patient's approach-oriented vicarious hope for events after his death: "I want to try and [make sure] … that [my family] all get on well together, and share everything together, like they do now…. And I love to see it, and I hope it continues, you know" (p. 145). The researchers construe this example as reflecting the patient's desire for an enduring legacy, the value the patient placed upon his family and his relationships with family members, and the effect such hope may have on the behaviour of family members. Similarly, based upon interviews focused upon end-of-life issues with 23 oncology patients, Eliott and Olver (2002) identify instances of hope *focused upon another* that contrast with instances of hope *focused upon the self*.

In longitudinal research, Herth (1990) conducted interviews with 30 terminally-ill adults, re-conducting interviews with a subset of them upon experiencing severe impairments in activities of daily living, and again when death appeared imminent. One of the interview questions asked, *What kind of things do you hope for*? Herth reports that with increasing levels of impairment, hope came to be focused on others more than on the self. For example, hope identified by respondents included: "happiness for my daughter and her new husband and family support for my wife" (p. 1254). These aims were summarized by one participant as "envisioning a positive outcome for those I love" (p. 1254). In open-ended interviews with 10 elderly palliative patients that included identifying things that gave them hope, Duggleby and Wright (2005) proffered evidence that hope transforms from a focus upon cure to a focus upon other outcomes including the welfare of others, as in the case of patients hoping for a better life in the future for their family.

Fanos et al. (2008) interviewed 16 adults diagnosed with Amyotrophic Lateral Sclerosis. The interview centered upon the meaning of hope to participants and ways to promote it. Eight hope themes emerged through content analysis of interview responses: hope for cure, social support, search for information, spiritual beliefs, adapting to changing capacities, living in the moment, self-transcendence, and limiting the impact on others. The latter two categories were relevant to other-oriented hope: 'Self-transcendence' included patients' desires to contribute to research in order to help future patients, while 'limiting the impact on others' included hoping that one's spouse would not be burdened too greatly as well as hoping that the disease would not strike one's grandchildren.

In a recent synthesis of this literature, Duggleby et al. (2012b) reviewed 20 qualitative studies focused upon experiences of hope among older adults with chronic illness. They identified several characteristics of hope among such individuals, including the multiple forms that hope can take. One type of co-existing hope identified by the researchers was *hope for their families* (p. 1217), suggesting the possibility that many chronically ill individuals transcend self-interest to incorporate the interests of close others. Similarly, in a review of 34 studies concerning hope among those in palliative care, Kylma et al. (2009) used content analysis to identify important aspects of patients' hope. A particular target of patients' hope was identified as hope directed toward the welfare of their family.

It is not only adults with illness who will direct their hope toward others. Hinds (1988) studied adolescent hopefulness, and changes in adolescent hopefulness as a function of illness status. Using a semistructured interview, including such questions as *What kinds of things do you hope for*? and *Tell me about a time when you felt very hopeful*, Hinds compared responses by healthy adolescents, those in a substance abuse recovery program, and those with various types of cancer. Four dimensions of hope emerged among the samples: taking a positive perspective; believing in personal possibilities; adopting a positive future orientation; and anticipating a positive personal future. Of greatest relevance to the current context, the group of adolescents with cancer yielded an additional hope dimension: *concern for and a focus on others*. Examples of the latter aspect of hope among those adolescents with cancer were: "others will not have to go through this illness"; "that there will be a cure soon so that patient 'x' will not die"; and "that my parents will be OK if I die" (p. 85). The author speculated that the directing of hope toward others by adolescents with cancer reflects a maturational process more typically seen among older adults. Based upon this author's research, hope is defined as "the degree to which adolescents possess a comforting or life-sustaining, reality-based belief that a positive future exists for themselves or others" (Hinds and Gattuso 1991, p. 92), placing other-oriented hope on par with self-oriented hope.

Similar findings emerged in a follow-up study by Hinds et al. (1999) in which 78 adolescents newly diagnosed with cancer completed a self-report measure of hopefulness *for self and others*, the 24-item Hopefulness Scale for Adolescents (Hinds and Gattuso 1991), and answered an interview question (*Please tell me what kinds of things you are hoping for now*). Results showed increasing self-reported hopefulness toward self and others across the four time periods (the rate of endorsement for self-oriented items versus other-oriented items was not separately reported by the authors). On the open-ended question, approximately 10–15 % of participants at each time period provided examples of hope toward others, such as "helping others by participating in research"; "having a safer and cleaner global environment"; and "stopping child abuse and other crimes" (p. 612).

## 4.6 Other-Oriented Hope Among Teachers

An older literature concerned the power of teacher expectancies on student performance (i.e., the effects of a teacher's optimism concerning the likely progress of particular students; Rosenthal 1991), but not of hope per se. Hope has been lamented as a neglected topic among education scholars (Edgoose 2010). Indeed, only a small number of brief references to other-oriented hope appear in the teaching literature. te Riele (2010) discusses the importance of hope held by teachers for their students. Duncan-Andrade (2009) discusses the crucial role of hope based in deep caring, love, and support provided by teachers to their students. Elbaz (1992) identifies teacher hopefulness for their students' outcomes as part of the moral aspect of teaching.

Only one piece of empirical work appears to have been conducted directly on vicarious hope among teachers. Larsen (2009) interviewed two Canadian university professors who specialized in counsellor education. Interviews centred on the professors' hope in relation to their academic careers. Both of the interviewees identified a central desire to contribute to others' lives, with the specific aim of benefitting others, including students and colleagues.

**Box 4.1: Hope-Focused Service Learning Examples**

Community service learning initiatives in schools provide obvious examples of an other-oriented focus. Community service learning (CSL) is especially designed to embed meaningful student learning within a community outreach context, often with the students themselves taking leadership in the projects undertaken. A program entitled *Hope-Focused Community Service Learning*, led by Dr. Lenora LeMay (LeMay 2013; LeMay et al. 2008) in a large mid-western Canadian city, has served as a fertile location for innovative hope-focused school programming in an ecologically embedded context. Working with Dr. LeMay, Ms. Regan Holt, a junior high school teacher, shares numerous stories of other-oriented hope she has witnessed in her students, stories within which both the 'hoper' and the 'receiver' appear to benefit. Teaching in an ethnically diverse inner city neighbourhood, many of Ms. Holt's junior high school students are newcomers to Canada, having arrived following truly harrowing circumstances in their countries of origin.

For many years, Ms. Holt has implemented a hope-focused service learning initiative in her classroom. The program usually begins with simple classroom exercises designed to invite the youth to reflect intentionally on their own experiences. Activities include a daily warm-up, low stakes, writing activity in 'hope scrapbooks'. Here, students are encouraged to write about whatever comes to mind when they think about hope. Responses often reflect whatever the students are experiencing both at home and even in the media. Common responses from the students are hopes concerning animals, including the fair treatment of zoo residents and even stray kittens found on the walk to school.

In time, the hope scrapbooking includes asking the students to describe a hopeful community. Ms. Holt's own hopes for her class are to build stronger community ties and reduce the apparent negative reputation surrounding youth in the neighbourhood. She also hopes that the students will act differently if they know others in their community better. Written responses from students have included numerous hopes for others in their community and ultimately lead to a community service activity, putting other-oriented hope into action. The class generates a plan. Previous classes have chosen activities such as cleaning up the playground, re-painting defaced playground benches, painting over graffiti in the neighbourhood, cleaning up broken glass, and making regular 'hope' visits to a nearby senior's residence.

In many ways the experience is transformational both for students and for the teacher. Ms. Holt begins by encouraging her students to imagine the world from another's perspective. In one example, students decided to reflect on what it would be like to walk through their neighbourhood as a very little child or an elderly person. From this, students articulated hopes for a safe and welcoming environment for the community's most vulnerable. They decided to repaint the playground benches, replacing graffiti with symbols of hope. When the benches were again defaced, the students returned to the benches to repaint and decorate them with hope. Indeed, even as they were repainting, adults walked by the school yard suggesting to the students that their efforts were futile, the benches likely only to be once more defaced. The students were polite but would have none of it. They hoped for something better for their community, they were willing to work for it, and they were willing to set a hopeful example for others.

In another large hope-focused project identified by one of Ms. Holt's classes, the students made a winter-time visit to a senior's residence directly across the street from their school. The students prepared to spend time with a senior and planned a craft activity they would complete together. Working one-on-one, each student was paired with an individual senior. Painting seasonally 'neutral' ornaments together, conversations ensued as they began to know one another. Completely unplanned, the students rather spontaneously decided to end their afternoon with the seniors by joining together in several rounds of Christmas carols. The activity surprised their teacher because the students represented numerous faiths, communities, and cultures. Though uninitiated by Ms. Holt, she took this spontaneous response as a distinct sign of other-oriented hope, a real respect by the students for the perspectives and hopes of the seniors.

## 4.7 General Instances of Other-Oriented Hope

Aside from the specific domains in which vicarious hope emerges in the research examples provided above, other studies have taken a broader view of the extent to which other-oriented hope occurs among people in general. The first substantial empirical support for general occurrences of other-oriented hope was proffered by Averill et al. (1990). In their Study 1, 150 American undergraduate participants were asked to provide an open-ended description of a past hope experience. Instructions further stipulated that the hope event not involve merely a want or a desire, and that it had occurred within the previous year. Students' descriptions of their recent hope experiences were subsequently grouped into four broad categories. The greatest number (41.3 %) of participants' hope descriptions were classifiable as achievement-related; the second largest category (25.3 %) contained hope pertaining to interpersonal relationships (e.g., romantic hopes); the third largest ("miscellaneous") category (24.7 %) concerned material objects such as desiring a new car; and, most important for the current purposes, the fourth and final category (8.7 %) reflected *altruistic hope* concerning the well-being of another person (e.g., hoping that a relative would recover from a serious illness). The hoped-for events were also rated by participants on their probability of occurrence, their importance, and their degree of personal versus situational control. Probability of attainment was stable across the four hope categories (around 60 % for all four). Importantly, participants with altruistic hope rated their hope as more important than the other groups. In distinction with the remaining hope categories, hope classified as altruistic was rated as having a higher degree of situational control as opposed to personal control. This study showed, first, that other-oriented hope occurs at a substantial rate among young adults, and that, despite being less common than self-oriented hope, other-oriented hope is rated as more important, less controllable, and of similar probability relative to self-oriented hope.

Further empirical support for the existence of other-oriented hope comes from the work (some of it reviewed in Chap. 1) of Bruininks and Malle (2005). In their second study, participants were asked to tell hope-related stories, which were contrasted with stories related to optimism, joy, wanting, or wishing. Fully 38 % of hope-related stories were categorized as altruistic in nature, typically concerning hope for positive outcomes of a close other. In contrast, only 11 and 10 % of stories generated as representative of optimism or joy were altruistic in nature, respectively, and none of the stories generated as representative of wanting or wishing were altruistic in nature. In sum, hope-related experiences were not infrequently other-oriented in nature, and were more often other-oriented in nature than experiences tied to different emotional states.

Howell et al. (in press) asked undergraduate students to *list 10 things for which you are hopeful*. Responses of participants were subsequently categorized as self- or other-oriented. Sixty-seven percent of participants generated at least one other-oriented hope statement (e.g., "That three of my family members can get past their sorrows"). Howell et al.'s study was unique in its inclusion of an experimental manipulation to prime the occurrence of vicarious hope, building upon the work of Gerbasi and Prentice (2013) in which other-interest was shown to be amenable to a priming manipulation. For a random half of participants in the Howell et al. study, the clause *for yourself or others* was included at the end of the instructional statement, as a prime for eliciting other-oriented hope. More participants generated at least one other-oriented hope when they were primed to consider others as the targets of their hope (85 %) compared to participants who were not so primed (67 %). This finding suggests that the frequency of other-oriented hope is amenable to change, such that future work could further explore both causes and consequences of more frequent other-oriented hope.

Ryff et al. (1994, see also 1996) had 215 parents of adult offspring respond to an open-ended question about hope they held for their children as the children grew up. The most frequently occurring hope identified by parents toward their children concerned happiness and educational success, followed by career success, establishing a happy family, experiencing personal fulfillment, being a good person, and having good health. Mothers and fathers identified similar hope for their children. In a quantitative portion of the same study, parents' ratings of their child's adjustment correlated positively with parental ratings of their own well-being. This suggests that if hope held by parents comes to be realized, parental well-being is likely to be relatively high. However, an additional finding was that parents who perceived that their child's current adjustment exceeded their own at the same age had significantly lower well-being, suggesting the possibility that if children's adjustment exceeds that hoped for by parents, parental well-being will be lower.

Lapierre et al. (2001) describe research on older individuals' life aspirations (as opposed to their hope per se). Respondents completed the Motivational Induction Method of Nuttin and Lens (1985), which involves finishing a series of sentence stems, such as "I would like…" and "I wish…". Responses are subsequently coded into several content categories. Most responses fell into the content categories labelled *self* (37.7 %) and *contact* (15.5 %). The third most common category was labelled *wishes for others* (9.5 %). Examples within the latter category included *That my son succeeds* and *That my husband will be cured*, showing that this category closely resembled other-oriented hope. Using these same content categories, Lapierre et al. (1993) report that *wishes for others* is a more frequent category among relatively younger elderly participants and among non-impaired relative to impaired participants. The authors suggest that less healthy individuals (i.e., relatively older and impaired) are more self-focused in their aspirations, emphasizing such fundamental goals as preserving their health.

As part of a larger study on middle-aged adults' perceptions of their futures, Newton et al. (2014) asked 155 adults, aged 55–58, about their hope for the future. Specifically, they were instructed to *Please describe your plans, dreams, or hopes for the future. What do you hope to accomplish in the future in your life story?* (p. 62). Each response was subsequently coded as to whether it reflected the self, others, or a composite of self and other themes. Results showed that 25 % of responses were other-oriented (e.g., help the homeless and help abused women), and 9 % reflected a composite of self- and other-orientation (e.g., publish another book that would help young women). An additional finding was that the frequency of other-oriented responses correlated positively with a measure of generativity; therefore, to the extent that middle-aged adults harboured other-oriented hope, they also experienced a somewhat greater sense of enriching the world for others.

Finally, Herth (1993) conducted semi-structured interviews with 60 older adults (age range of 60–100). Six questions concerning hope were posed to participants, including the open-ended question *What kinds of things do you hope for?* Herth identified changes as a function of age and impairment level of respondents, with those older than 80 and experiencing mild to moderate impairment being more likely to harbour hope focused on others compared to those who were higher functioning. Moreover, those living in long-term care facilities with moderate to severe impairment directed their hope almost entirely toward others. Summarizing participants' responses to the question *What does hope mean to you?*, Herth states, "Hope is an inner power that facilitates the transcendence of the present situation and enables a reality based expectation of a brighter tomorrow for self and/or others" (p. 146). In conjunction with the definition of hope proffered by Hinds and Gattuso (1991) described above, Herth's is only the second published definition of hope that includes a direct reference to other-oriented hope.

In sum, a significant amount of empirical evidence has accrued over the last two decades of hope research that supports the concept of other-oriented hope. The evidence comes from specific domains of life experiences, such as parenting a severely ill child, but it also comes from more general circumstances, such as simply listing hopes for the future as an undergraduate student. Adolescents and a broad age range of adults, including those from various countries and cultures, have provided evidence and examples of vicarious hope. Notably, much of the evidence has accrued indirectly, emerging in research that did not necessarily set-out to unearth other-oriented hope; thus, other-oriented hope emerged independently of researchers' direct elicitation of it. Quantitative, qualitative, and mixed-method research approaches have yielded evidence of other-oriented hope; such converging findings across divergent methods speak to the robust nature of the phenomenon of other-oriented hope. Finally, a number of syntheses of qualitative studies have yielded consistent evidence of other-oriented hope.

## References


Amendolia, B. (2010). Hope and parents of the critically ill newborn. *Advances in Neonatal Care, 10*, 140–144.

Austin, W., Brintnell, E. S., Goble, E., Kagan, L., Kreitzer, L., Larsen, D. J., & Leier, B. (2013). *Lying down in the ever-falling snow: Canadian health professionals' experience of compassion fatigue*. Waterloo, Ontario: Wilfred Laurier University Press.

Averill, J. R., Catlin, G., & Chon, K. K. (1990). *Rules of hope*. New York: Springer.

Bamforth, S., & Pederson, A. (2008). Hope, recovery and schizophrenia: The experience of caring and coping. Available at http://www.murdoch.edu.au/School-of-Psychology-and-Exercise-Science/Research/Psychology-Research/Hope-recovery-and-schizophrenia-The-experience-of-caring-and-coping/.

Bland, R., & Darlington, Y. (2002). The nature and sources of hope: Perspectives of family caregivers of people with serious mental illness. *Perspectives in Psychiatric Care, 38*, 61–68.

Bruininks, P., & Malle, B. F. (2005). Distinguishing hope from optimism and related affective states. *Motivation and Emotion, 29*, 327–355.

Cohn, E., Miller, L. J., & Tickle-Degnen, L. (2000). Parental hopes for therapy outcomes: Children with sensory modulation disorders. *American Journal of Occupational Therapy, 54*, 36–43.

Coppock, T. E., Owen, J. J., Zagarskas, E., & Schmidt, M. (2010). The relationship between therapist and client hope with therapy outcomes. *Psychotherapy Research, 20*, 619–626.

Darlington, Y., & Bland, B. (1999). Strategies for encouraging and maintaining hope among people living with serious mental illness. *Australian Social Work, 52*, 17–23.

Dufrane, K., & Leclair, S. W. (1984). Using hope in the counseling process. *Counseling and Values, 29*, 32–41.

Duggleby, W., Bally, J., Cooper, D., Doell, H., & Thomas, R. (2012a). Engaging hope: The experiences of male spouses of women with breast cancer. *Oncology Nursing Forum, 39*, 400–406.

Duggleby, W., Hicks, D., Nekolaichuk, C., Holtslander, L., Williams, A., Chambers, T., & Eby, J. (2012b). Hope, older adults, and chronic illness: A metasynthesis of qualitative research. *Journal of Advanced Nursing, 68*, 1211–1223.

Duggleby, W., Holtslander, L., Kylma, J., Duncan, V., Hammond, C., & Williams, A. (2010). Metasynthesis of the hope experience of family caregivers of persons with chronic illness. *Qualitative Health Research, 20*, 148–158.

Duggleby, W., Schroeder, D., & Nekolaichuk, C. (2013). Hope and connection: The experience of family caregivers of persons with dementia living in a long term care facility. *BMC Geriatrics, 13*, 1–8.

Duggleby, W., Williams, A., Holtslander, L., Cunningham, S., & Wright, K. (2011). The chaos of caregiving and hope. *Qualitative Social Work, 11*, 459–469.

Duggleby, W., Williams, A., Wright, K., & Bollinger, S. (2009). Renewing everyday hope: The hope experience of family caregivers of persons with dementia. *Issues in Mental Health Nursing, 30*, 514–521.

Duggleby, W., & Wright, K. (2005). Transforming hope: How elderly palliative patients live with hope. *Canadian Journal of Nursing Research, 37*, 70–84.

Duncan-Andrade, J. M. R. (2009). Note to educators: Hope required when growing roses in concrete. *Harvard Educational Review, 79*, 181–194.

Edgoose, J. (2010). Hope in the unexpected: How can teachers still make a difference in the world? *Teachers College Record, 112*, 386–406.

Elbaz, F. (1992). Hope, attentiveness, and caring for difference: The moral voice in teaching. *Teaching and Teaching Education, 8*, 421–432.

Eliott, J. A., & Olver, I. N. (2002). The discursive properties of "hope": A qualitative analysis of cancer patients' speech. *Qualitative Health Research, 12*, 173–193.

Eliott, J. A., & Olver, I. N. (2007). Hope and hoping in the talk of dying cancer patients. *Social Science and Medicine, 64*, 138–149.

Eliott, J. A., & Olver, I. N. (2009). Hope, life, and death: A qualitative analysis of dying cancer patients' talk about hope. *Death Studies, 33*, 609–638.

Fanos, J. H., Gelinas, D. F., Foster, R. S., Postone, N., & Miller, R. G. (2008). Hope in palliative care: From narcissism to self-transcendence in Amyotrophic Lateral Sclerosis. *Journal of Palliative Medicine, 11*, 470–475.

Faso, D. J., Neal-Beevers, A. R., & Carlson, C. L. (2013). Vicarious futurity, hope, and well-being in parents of children with autism spectrum disorder. *Research in Autism Spectrum Disorders, 7*, 288–297.

Flaskas, C. (2007). Holding hope and hopelessness: Therapeutic engagements with the balance of hope. *Journal of Family Therapy, 29*, 186–202.

Flesaker, K., & Larsen, D. (2010). To offer hope you must have hope: Accounts of hope for reintegration counsellors working with women on parole and probation. *Qualitative Social Work, 11*, 61–79.

Frank, J. D. (1968). The role of hope in psychotherapy. *International Journal of Psychiatry, 5*, 383–395.

Freidman-Yakoobian, M. S., de Mamani, A. W., & Mueser, K. T. (2009). Predictors of distress and hope in relatives of individuals with schizophrenia. *International Psychiatry and Related Sciences, 46*, 130–140.

Gadgeel, S. M. (2011). Hope and realism: The perfect balance? *Journal of Clinical Oncology, 16*, 2291–2292.

Gebhardt, C., McGehee, L. A., Grindel, C. G., & Testani-Dufour, L. (2011). Caregiver and nurse hopes for recovery of patients with acquired brain injury. *Rehabilitation Nursing, 36*, 3–12.

Gerbasi, M. E., & Prentice, D. A. (2013). The self- and other-interest inventory. *Journal of Personality and Social Psychology, 105*, 495–514.

Godfrey, J. J. (1987). *A philosophy of human hope*. Dordrecht: Martinus Nijhoff Publishers.

Hernandez, M., Barrio, C., & Yamada, A.-M. (2013). Hope and burden among Latino families of adults with schizophrenia. *Family Process, 52*, 697–708.

Herth, K. (1990). Fostering hope in terminally-ill people. *Journal of Advanced Nursing, 13*, 1250–1259.

Herth, K. (1993). Hope in older adults in community and institutional settings. *Issues in Mental Health Nursing, 14*, 139–156.

Hinds, P. S. (1988). Adolescent hopefulness in illness and health. *Advances in Nursing Science, 10*, 79–88.

Hinds, P. S., & Gattuso, J. (1991). Measuring hopefulness in adolescents. *Journal of Pediatric Oncology Nursing, 8*, 92–94.

Hinds, P. S., Quargnenti, A., Fairclough, D., Bush, A. J., Betcher, D., Rissmiller, G., et al. (1999). Hopefulness and its characteristics in adolescents with cancer. *Western Journal of Nursing Research, 21*, 600–616.

Holtslander, L. F., & Duggleby, W. D. (2009). The hope experience of older bereaved women who cared for a spouse with terminal cancer. *Qualitative Health Research, 19*, 388–400.

Holtslander, L., Duggleby, W., Williams, A. W., & Wright, K. (2005). The experience of hope for informal caregivers of palliative patients. *Journal of Palliative Care, 21*(4), 285–292.

Howell, A., Bailie, T., & Buro, K. (in press). Evidence for vicarious hope and vicarious gratitude. *Journal of Happiness Studies.*

Jevne, R. F. (1991). *It all begins with hope: Patients, caregivers, and the bereaved speak out*. San Diego, CA: LuraMedia.

Karanci, A. N. (1995). Caregivers of Turkish schizophrenic patients: Causal attributions, burdens and attitudes to help from the health care professionals. *Social Psychiatry and Psychiatric Epidemiology, 30*, 261–268.

Kausar, S., Jevne, R. F., & Sobsey, D. (2003). Hope in families of children with developmental disabilities. *Journal on Developmental Disabilities, 10*, 35–46.

Kelly, A. (2007). Hope is forked: Hope, loss, treatments, and AIDS dementia. *Qualitative Health Research, 17*, 866–872.

Kirpalani, H. M., Parkin, P. C., Willian, A. R., Fehlings, D. L., Rosenbaum, P. L., King, D., & Van Nie, A. J. (2000). Quality of life in spina bifida: Importance of parental hope. *Archives of Disorders in Childhood, 83*, 293–307.

Koenig, T., & Spano, R. (2007). The cultivation of social workers' hope in personal life and professional practice. *Journal of Religion and Spirituality in Social Work, 26*, 45–61.

Kopelowicz, A., Zarate, R., Gonzalez Smith, V., Mintz, J., & Liberman, R. P. (2003). Disease management in Latinos with schizophrenia: A family-assisted, skills training approach. *Schizophrenia Bulletin, 29*, 211–227.

Kylma, J., Duggleby, W., Cooper, D., & Molander, G. (2009). Hope in palliative care: An integrative review. *Palliative and Supportive Care, 7*, 365–377.

Kylma, J., & Juvakka, T. (2007). Hope in parents of adolescents with cancer: Factors endangering and engendering parental hope. *European Journal of Oncology Nursing, 11*, 262–271.

Kylma, J., Juvakka, T., Nikkonen, M., Korhonen, T., & Isohanni, M. (2006). Hope and schizophrenia: An integrative review. *Journal of Psychiatric and Mental Health Nursing, 13*, 651–664.

Lapierre, S., Bouffard, L., & Bastin, E. (1993). Motivational goal objects in later life. *International Journal of Aging and Human Development, 45*, 287–303.

Lapierre, S., Bouffard, L., Dube, M., Labelle, R., & Bastin, E. (2001). Aspirations and well-being in old age. In P. Schmuck & K. M. Sheldon (Eds.), *Life goals and well-being: Towards a positive psychology of human striving* (pp. 102–115).

Larsen, D. J. (2009). "It gives me a kind of grounding": Two university educators' narratives of hope in worklife. In A. M. A. Mattos (Ed.), *Narratives on teaching and teacher education: An international perspective* (pp. 151–166). New York: Palgrave Macmillan.

Larsen, D. J., Stege, R., Edey, W., & Ewasiw, J. (2014). Working with unrealistic or unshared hope in the counselling session. *British Journal of Guidance and Counselling*. doi:10.1080/03069885.2014.895798.

Larsen, D. J., Stege, R., & Flesaker, K. (2013). 'It's important for me not to let go of hope': Psychologists' in-session experiences of hope. *Reflective Practice: International and Multidisciplinary Perspectives, 14*, 472–486.

Larson, E. (1998). Reframing the meaning of disability to families: The embrace of paradox. *Social Science and Medicine, 47*, 865–875.

LeMay, L. (2013). A narrative inquiry into teachers' experiences of working with hope. Unpublished doctoral dissertation. University of Alberta, Edmonton, AB.

LeMay, L., Edey, W., & Larsen, D. (2008). *Nurturing hopeful souls: Practices and activities for working with children and youth*. Edmonton, AB: Hope Foundation of Alberta.

Manrique, J. F. D. (1984). Hope as a means of therapy in the work of Karen Horney. *American Journal of Psychoanalysis, 44*, 301–310.

Newton, N. J., Herr, J. M., Pollack, J. I., & McAdams, D. P. (2014). Selfless or selfish? Generativity and narcissism as components of legacy. *Journal of Adult Development, 21*, 59–68.

Nuttin, J., & Lens, W. (1985). *Future time perspective and motivation: Theory and research method*. Hillsdale, NJ: Erlbaum.

Patel, C. T. C. (1996). Hope-inspiring strategies of spouses of critically ill adults. *Journal of Holistic Nursing, 14*, 44–65.

Pellegrino, E. D., & Thomasma, D. C. (1996). *The Christian virtues in medical practice*. Washington, DC: Georgetown University Press.

Redlich, D., Hadas-Lidor, N., Weiss, P., & Amirav, I. (2010). Mediated learning experience intervention increases hope of family members coping with a relative with severe mental illness. *Community Mental Health Journal, 46*, 409–415.

Richardson, K., MacLeod, R., & Kent, B. (2012). A Steinian approach to an empathic understanding of hope among patients and clinicians in the culture of palliative care. *Journal of Advanced Nursing, 68*, 686–694.

Rosenthal, R. (1991). Teaching expectancy effects: A brief update 25 years after the Pygmalion experiment. *Journal of Research in Education, 1*, 3–12.

Ryff, C. D., Lee, Y. H., Essex, M. J., & Schmutte, P. S. (1994). My children and me: Midlife evaluations of grown children and of self. *Psychology and Aging, 9*, 195–205.

Ryff, C. D., Schmutte, P. S., & Lee, Y. H. (1996). How children turn out: Implications for parental self-evaluation. In. C. D. Ryff & M. M. Seltzer (Eds.), *The parental experience in midlife* (pp. 383–422). University of Chicago Press.

Simpson, C. (2004). When hope makes us vulnerable: A discussion of patient-healthcare provider interactions in the context of hope. *Bioethics, 18*, 428–447.

Snyder, C. R., Michael, S. T., & Cheavens, J. S. (1999). Hope as a psychotherapeutic foundation of common factors, placebos, and expectancies. In M. A. Hubble, B. L. Duncan, & S. D. Miller (Eds.), *The heart and soul of change: What works in therapy* (pp. 179–200). Washington, DC, USA: American Psychological Association.

Stein, C. H., Mann, L. M., & Hunt, M. G. (2007). Ever onward: The personal strivings of young adults coping with serious mental illness and the hopes of their parents. *American Journal of Orthopsychiatry, 77*, 104–112.

te Riele, K. (2010). Philosophy of hope: Concepts and applications for working with marginalised youth. *Journal of Youth Studies, 13*, 35–46.

Thorne, S. (2008). *Interpretive description*. Walnut Creek, CA: Left Coast Press.

Tibaldi, G., & Govers, L. (2012). Evidence-based hope for recovery from "schizophrenia": A common objective for all stakeholders in the mental health field. *Psychosis: Psychological, Social, and Integrative Approaches, 4*. doi:10.1080/17522439.2011.584349.

Truitt, M., Biesecker, B., Capone, G., Bailey, T., & Erby, L. (2012). The role of hope in adaptation to uncertainty: The experience of caregivers of children with Down syndrome. *Patient Education and Counseling, 87*, 233–238.

Verhaeghe, S. T. L., Van Zuuren, F. J., Defloor, T., Duijnstee, M. S. H., & Grypdonck, M. H. F. (2007). How does information influence hope in family members of traumatic coma patients in intensive care unit? *Journal of Clinical Nursing, 16*, 1488–1497.

Weingarten, K. (2010). Reasonable hope: Construct, clinical applications, and supports. *Family Process, 49*, 5–25.

Wildes, K. (1999). Hope: A necessary virtue for health care. *Bioethics Forum, 15*, 25–29.

Wong, M. G., & Heriot, S. A. (2007). Vicarious futurity in autism and childhood dementia. *Journal of Autism and Developmental Disorders, 37*, 1833–1841.

Wong, M. G., & Heriot, S. A. (2008). Parents of children with cystic fibrosis: How they hope, cope, and despair. *Child: Care Health, and Development, 34*, 344–354.

# Chapter 5
# Origins and Consequences of Other-Oriented Hope, and Theoretical Frameworks Relevant to Its Understanding

## 5.1 General

*...I pass over myself and meet the other in his or her true otherness, an otherness that is irreducible to me or to my own interests in the world.*
—van Manen 2002, p. 270

*Wishing: in gladness and in safety,*
*may all things be at ease*
—The Buddha's words on lovingkindness (*Metta Sutta*)

In this chapter, we examine psychological and situational influences on other-oriented hope, we examine several consequences, both beneficial and detrimental, of other-oriented hope, and we examine theoretical frameworks pertinent to other-oriented hope and which situate other-oriented hope within broader, more encompassing perspectives on a life well-lived.

## 5.2 Origins of Other-Oriented Hope

In this section, we examine distal and then more proximal influences on the development of other-oriented hope. Unfortunately, there is little direct research or theorizing on this topic; as a result, our consideration of the causes of other-oriented hope is often speculative, and rests mostly upon findings and arguments concerning related phenomena.

Eisenberg (2002) reviewed evidence for parental influences on the development of empathy-related responding and of prosocial behaviour, which may be pertinent to identifying influences on other-oriented hope. Eisenberg identifies the *authoritative parental style* as conducive to the development of empathy-related responding in children. This is a warm-but-firm style of parenting in which, for example, a parent sets clear expectations and limits, but does so in the context of a loving, close, and caring parent-child relationship. This style of parenting can be



A.J. Howell and D.J. Larsen, *Understanding Other-Oriented Hope*,
SpringerBriefs in Well-Being and Quality of Life Research,
DOI 10.1007/978-3-319-15007-9_5

contrasted with an *authoritarian* style (i.e., firm but not warm) and with a *permissive* style (i.e., warm but not firm), both of which have been shown to be less related to a child's level of empathy.

Other socialization influences identified by Eisenberg (2002) as conducive to empathy-related responding include appropriate modeling of emotion regulation, establishing a secure attachment, and parental use of reasoning or inductive explanations for caring about others. Eisenberg also identifies several parental influences conducive to prosocial behaviour, including modeling of prosocial behaviour, reinforcement of prosocial behaviour, and socialization of prosocial values such as benevolence. We speculate here that these early socialization practices may instill a tendency to experience other-oriented hope, reflecting the fact that the latter can also involve both empathic feelings and caring behaviour toward others.

Distal, or background, influences on the development of other-oriented hope may also include cultural practices. Pertinent to this issue is the distinction between collectivistic and individualistic cultures; that is, cultures in which people are, respectively, relatively more or less reliant upon and concerned about close others (Triandis et al. 1988). Research on hope itself now traverses various cultures. Examples include Averill et al.'s (1990) research examining the meaning of hope in both Korea and the United States; Mattos' (2009) research on the role of hope in teaching practices in Brazil; and Cherrington's (2013) research with indigenous youth in South Africa. Across cultures, hope is consistently identified as an important concept and human experience, while the attributes of hope appear to vary somewhat based on cultural context. For example, working within an indigenous context, Cherrington identifies hope as a collective or community phenomenon, focusing on the notion of 'we hope' rather than 'I hope'. It may be that other-oriented hope is cultivated and understood differently within collectivistic cultures than individualistic cultures, given the emphasis within the former on one's relatedness to others, especially to kin and other members of one's community. Indeed, the focus within individualistic cultures on personal agency and uniqueness may mitigate the development of high levels of other-oriented hope and encourage, instead, a focus upon one's own future attainments and achievements.

Proximal influences on other-oriented hope can include both those that reside within individuals and those that reflect the immediate social context. Personality traits directly related to one's relatedness to others—such as agreeableness, empathy, and compassion—should conduce toward other-oriented hope. Having a strong need for belongingness or relatedness to others would auger well for the development of other-oriented hope. Endorsing social values such as benevolence and universalism would also be conducive to holding hope for others, as would construing oneself as interdependent with others as opposed to independent of others. The possession of these traits likely reflects both early socialization experiences, such as those described above, and genetic influences as evidenced by the heritability of personality dispositions such as agreeableness.

Outside of those personal characteristics that are directly related to propelling people toward others, other characteristics may also be germane to the development of other-oriented hope. Mindfulness, or the ability to sustain a state of awareness, attention, and nonjudgmental acceptance, may be an important contributor to other-oriented hope. Mindfulness may increase one's ability to notice, attend to, and accept others' aspirations and therefore to come to hold similar aspirations for others' futures (e.g., Harvey et al. 2002; Weingarten 2010). The characteristic of humility may incline people to be more focused upon another's future than on their own. And, having a strong sense of fairness may compel people to hope for just outcomes concerning another's plight.

Close familial, romantic, and companionate relationships will likely conduce toward other-oriented hope. Other-oriented hope is expected to most often be directed toward those closest to us, such as our parents, siblings, partners, and long-standing friends (e.g., Howell et al. in press). According to Batson and Shaw (1991), greater motivation to improve the welfare of close others reflects greater empathy toward those to whom we are emotionally attached. Professional and social roles may also influence the extent to which other-oriented hope is experienced; specifically, the roles of parent, caregiver, health care provider, psychotherapist, coach, or teacher may foster the frequent occurrence of other-oriented hope relative to roles or occupations that are less inclusive of a significant caring or nurturing element.

There may be developmental and gender influences on other-oriented hope. It is likely that hope is more egocentric at younger ages and more other-oriented at older ages. Recall the research of Herth (1993), who showed that very old individuals expressed the greatest degree of other-oriented hope. In a related domain, Van Lange et al. (2007) showed that the proportion of people whose social value orientation was classifiable as *prosocial* increased with age, whereas the proportion classifiable as *individualistic* or *competitive* decreased with age. Turning to gender, it is possible that females, on average, will engage in a greater degree of other-oriented hope than will males, given evidence (albeit mixed) of gender differences in related domains such as empathic responding (Eisenberg and Lennon 1983).

**Box 5.1: Annie's Song**

Little research has examined the development, experience, and role of hope in childhood, especially as these relate to other-oriented hope. Nevertheless, our experience suggests that the seeds of these fundamental aspects of human experience are likely sown in very early life. As a counselling psychologist, I (D. L.) remember working for a lengthy period of time with a family whose baby son began his life in the neonatal intensive care unit. The young boy's life was fragile and he lived in and out of the children's hospital for many of his early years. His life and future were often in serious question. The family lived a disrupted existence, commuting to hospital from their rural home for months at a time. Their daughter, Annie, a three year old, took the lifestyle and the worry for her little brother as one of life's givens.

Sometime after her brother's birth, I asked Annie whether she knew anything about hope. Annie was a precocious four year-old, and I remember the conversation vividly because its depth surprised me:

"Do you know anything about hope, Annie?" A good question, I thought, because closed questions are generally easier for children to answer.

"Yup", Annie chirped.

"Do you want to tell me about it?" Another good closed question, I thought.

"Nope", Annie replied as cheerfully. Oh dear, I thought. Here is where closed questions can cause problems. Where to from here? As quick as these thoughts race through my mind, Annie continued.

"But I could sing you a song about it!"

"I would love to hear it!"

Annie sang a very long and lovely song, one she made up on the spot. The details of the 'verses' are lost to me now but the refrain still arrests.

Over and over she sang in her little girl voice, "Hope is a band-aid of love. Hope is a band-aid of love. Hope is a band-aid of love …".

Annie told me about hope, other-oriented hope in the way that children communicate, through the arts, song, image, metaphor.

When I asked Annie's mom about the song, she responded without hesitation. "That song is about me. She is hoping for me."

Situational influences on other-oriented hope also require consideration. The research reviewed in Chap. 4 strongly points to the element of vulnerability in another person as a situational influence on other-oriented hope. Learning about others' vulnerability likely triggers compassion or empathy which, in turn, elicits other-oriented hope. In unpublished research, Bailie (2014) showed that the induction of compassion led to a higher frequency of other-oriented hope. In addition to other-oriented hope occurring in response to another's vulnerability, vicarious hope appears also to be triggered by one's own vulnerability. Chapter 4 reviewed research showing that as people reach the end of their lives, a greater proportion of their hopes come to be other-oriented (e.g., Eliott and Olver 2007; Herth 1990, 1993).

Additional situational elements include contextual differences such as cooperative versus competitive environments. Perhaps other-oriented hope flows more freely in classrooms or societal settings in which cooperativeness with others is expected and reinforced; in contrast, other-oriented hope may flow less freely in those *dog-eat-dog* settings in which competition with others is common, expected, and encouraged. *Jigsaw classrooms*, in which children cooperate with each other in order to complete various assignments (Aronson and Patnoe 1997), may have the impact of increasing other-oriented hope.

Additional situational elements germane to other-oriented hope include perceiving the other's goal attainment as valuable and as possible; without such perceptions, other-oriented hope would be unnecessary or unrealistic, respectively. Finally, the priming or activation of an other-oriented mindset may temporarily increase other-oriented hope, as in the research by Howell et al. (in press) reviewed in Chap. 4. In that study, the rate of other-oriented hope increased when participants were subtly reminded that their hope could concern themselves or others, relative to the condition in which no such reminder was given. Presumably, the activation of a self-oriented mindset, perhaps via reminding people of their unique characteristics that make them stand apart, would have the opposite effect on other-oriented hope. Therefore, recently activated mental states may temporarily orient a person to experience other-oriented hope to a greater or lesser degree.

## 5.3 Benefits and Costs of Other-Oriented Hope

There are several potential adaptive consequences to the holding of hope for others. From an instrumental viewpoint, vicarious hope may be seen as producing beneficial outcomes for the hopeful person, for those who are the targets of their hope, and for the relationship between the parties. Hope is well-established as a psychological asset, with numerous benefits associated with hope for both physical and mental health outcomes (e.g., Snyder 2002). Hopeful people are happier and healthier than less hopeful people. By extrapolation, it is likely the case that those whose hope is often other-oriented may, too, experience these benefits. Indeed, there is evidence that the correlates (and possibly benefits) of being hopeful toward others include reduced stress (Faso et al. 2013; Hernandez et al. 2013; Kopelowicz et al. 2003; Wong and Heriot 2008). This suggests the possibility that when parents hope for their ill child, when social workers hope for their struggling clients, or when terminally ill individuals extend their hope outward toward loved ones, the stress and strain surrounding such challenging situations is lessened. In line with Lazarus (1999) view of hope as an emotion-focused coping strategy, holding hope for others may be a way of regulating one's emotional composure in trying situations.

Bovens (1999) identifies several additional benefits associated with hope. These include the function of hope in helping to realize desired outcomes and in reducing risk aversion. That is, when hopeful, individuals are more motivated to pursue their aspirations and are less likely to postpone or inhibit their goal pursuit due to fear of failure or other concerns. The enabling, engaging function of hope and its counteraction of risk aversion may apply quite directly to other-oriented hope; that is, to the degree that other-oriented hope motivates action toward the attainment of hoped-for outcomes, the likelihood of reaching those endpoints is increased. Hoping that a friend does well on an upcoming exam may facilitate that very outcome, such as by encouraging the friend to study, not offering alternative activities to the friend that would interfere with goal attainment, not dwelling upon the threat of failing or exaggerating the consequences of such an outcome, and providing affirming feedback along the way. In related work, Hollis et al. (2007)

discuss *borrowed* hope; for those with no hope, others who have hope for them can be impactful, because hope can be viewed as 'contagious'.

In addition to benefitting both the bearer and the recipient of other-oriented hope, other-oriented hope may have significant interpersonal benefits in the form of relationship enhancement. To the extent that the person targeted by vicarious hope is appreciative of that form of attention, recognition, and support, the relationship between the two parties may be substantially enhanced. Indeed, people who express hope for their partner's future success are strengthening their relationship with that partner in a manner similar to the effects of an *active-constructive* style of response to another's past success. Active-constructing responding characterizes a person's supportive and celebratory response to a positive event experienced and disclosed by a partner. Active-constructive responses occur as part of the capitalization process, wherein a person shares positive news with a partner and thereby *capitalizes upon* the experience (Gable and Reis 2010; Langston 1994). Research by Gable et al. (2004, 2006) showed that active-constructive responses to another's act of capitalization, as opposed to passive and destructive responses, are associated with adaptive consequences for the disclosing individual and for the relationship. Such effects may also follow acts of other-oriented hope, which differ from acts of active-constructive responding primarily on the basis of their temporal orientation: the celebration of past successes in the case of active-constructive responding and the anticipation of future successes in the case of other-oriented hope. Indeed, borrowing from the concept of active-constructive responding, other-oriented hope can be viewed as an active, constructive form of future-oriented thinking toward others which may carry similar adaptive benefits as those attached to responding in an active-constructive manner to others' past and present accomplishments.

In addition to its instrumental functions in generating extrinsic benefits for the bearer and the target of other-oriented hope, and for the relationship between those two parties, there may be properties of other-oriented hope that provide intrinsic reinforcement for its experience and expression. Bovens (1999) identifies several inherent, *built-in* values associated with hope, including pleasures of anticipation, increased self-understanding, and loving relationships. These benefits of hoping cannot be separated from the process of hoping itself; they are intrinsically wedded to it. Each of these intrinsic values associated with hope may be associated also with other-oriented hope; indeed, Bovens makes explicit reference to other-oriented hope in underscoring the association between hope and loving relationships. The remaining two intrinsic values identified by Bovens would also appear to accompany other-oriented hope: it is pleasurable to anticipate the attainment of positive outcomes of another, and we stand a high likelihood of learning something about ourselves when we engage in other-oriented hope. In relation to this latter point, McGeer (2004) argues that the experience of hoping for others may allow people to clarify their own hope:

> Thus, in caring for the clarity of others' hopes and hopeful initiatives, we engage more readily in a practice of reflection and analysis for them, which often has consequences for the way we think about ourselves. (p. 124)

Thus, by attending to the nature of the hope we harbour for others, we glean insight into our own values, aspirations, and priorities. McGeer also identifies social feedback processes which allow other-oriented hope to facilitate self-oriented hope:

> Hoping well thus involves cultivating a meta-disposition in which some of one's hopeful energy becomes directed toward supporting the hopeful agency of others and, hence, toward creating the kind of environment in which one's own hopeful energy is supplemented by the hopeful energy renewed in them. (p. 123)

A 'virtuous cycle' of hope may be ignited when one's hope for others inspires those others, whose hope in turn gets directed back to regenerate hope for oneself. Of course, people other than the original bearer of other-oriented hope may come to benefit from the boosted hopefulness of the recipient. In addition, other-oriented hope may facilitate commitment on behalf of those carrying such hope to persevere in their own circumstances in order to bear witness to potential realization of vicarious hope; thus, other-oriented hope may induce a general motivated state of engagement or vitality.

Just as there are numerous positive consequences of vicarious hope, other-oriented hope may also be associated with costs or drawbacks, and these may pertain to the self, the other, and the relationship between self and other. Similar to recognized drawbacks or risks of self-oriented hope, other-oriented hope may be associated with a failure to accept things the way they are, frustration upon hope being dashed, risk taking, or the failure to limit losses (Bovens 1999; Lazarus 1991). Given the lower controllability of other-oriented hope compared to self-oriented hope (Averill et al. 1990; see also Day 1969), one may expend time and energy in holding and acting on hope toward others that ultimately bear little fruit. There is also an *opportunity-cost* to other-oriented hope: Time spent hoping for another is time *not* spent generating, contemplating, or acting toward either one's own hope or to yet other people's hope. As an example, the parent who places all hope on a child thereby neglects their own aspirations, curtailing opportunities for personal growth and achievement and the psychological gains attached to such self-oriented pursuits.

There may be costs to the recipient of other-oriented hope in the form of feeling coerced or controlled by others whose vicarious hope is not shared by the recipient. Therefore, some forms of other-oriented hope may reveal only the desired outcomes of the hoping agent as opposed to the person to whom the hope applies. In the classic example, a parent's hope for a child may not be hope that is held by the child him- or herself, and therefore may be experienced as a significant source of undue pressure and stress by the child. Such coercive hope is, in turn, likely to be harmful to the relationship between the person harbouring the other-oriented hope and the target of that hope. Li and Larsen (2012) offer a telling example of parental hope impacting children. In a narrative study of two Chinese youth sent for a Canadian education at an early age (14 and 16), Li and Larsen inquired into experiences of adjustment and hope for these girls. Seeing Canada as a land of opportunity to learn English and gain a better education, the journeys for both adolescents to Canada were spawned by hope. However, vastly different narratives unfolded. At 14, Lan was told by her family to travel to Canada; her story is characterized by sadness and isolation. In largest measure, she was living her parents' hope but not her own. She eventually found her own sources of hope in Canada but the road was exceedingly painful. In contrast, when she was 16 years old, Peony approached her father asking to study in Canada. She had her own hopes about what a Canadian education would mean for her future. Reluctantly, her parents agreed. Though the transition was difficult, Peony's story is largely one of satisfaction in learning to live out her own hope.

In another context, Beste (2005) expresses concern over medical staff "projecting an end … that patients may not even embrace, and …. depriving them of meaningful self-determination" (p. 227; see also Simpson 2004). Offering an antidote to autonomy-negating hope, McGeer (2004) uses the term *scaffolding* to characterize the optimal degree of hope-related respect, recognition, and support given to others. In effective scaffolding, "individuals are naturally drawn into a kind of community of mutually responsive hope in which each person's hopes become partly invested in the hopeful agency of others and vice versa" (McGeer 2004, p. 118). Similarly, Larsen et al.'s (2013) notion of *empathic hoping*, in which the target's hope is mirrored by the other, may be a particularly adaptive form of other-oriented hope, circumventing the danger of imposing hope on the other.

In an extreme form, other-oriented hope bears resemblance to *other-oriented perfectionism*. Hewitt and Flett (2004) argue that perfectionism can be directed toward the self or others. In the former case, perfectionism involves expectations placed upon oneself for unreasonably high performance, whereas in the latter case, perfectionism involves expecting others to uphold an unreasonably high standard and expressing criticism when others fail to meet this expectation. It is possible that other-oriented hope occasionally takes the form of other-oriented expectations for perfection. For example, a parent may *hope* that a child performs well in school, but this could take the form of an overly demanding standard of achievement that is difficult or impossible for the child to attain, creating distress in the child's life and conflict within the parent-child relationship.

Stoeber (2014) studied the relationship of other-oriented perfectionism and self-oriented perfectionism to social goal setting; negative traits of narcissism, Machiavellianism, and psychopathy; and positive traits of honesty-humility and altruism. Measures of each of these constructs were given to a large number of undergraduate student participants. Other-oriented perfectionism was measured with items such as, *If I do not set very high standards for people I know, they are likely to end up second-rate people* and *If I scold others for their failure to live up to expectations, it will help them in the future*. Self-oriented perfectionism was assessed with items such as *I demand nothing less than perfection of myself*. Results showed that higher other-oriented perfectionism was associated with lower adoption of nurturance and intimacy goals (i.e., goals of making others feel good and getting closer to others, respectively), whereas higher self-oriented perfectionism was associated with higher adoption of these goals. Other-oriented perfectionism was associated with greater narcissism, Machiavellianism, and psychopathy, whereas self-oriented perfectionism was associated with lower Machiavellianism and psychopathy. Finally, other-oriented perfectionism was associated with lower altruism and honesty-humility, whereas self-oriented perfection was associated with greater altruism. As a whole, other-oriented perfectionism was associated with detrimental attributes, especially attributes concerning one's ability to relate to others in a positive fashion. As summarized by Stoeber, "Other-oriented perfectionism appears to be an ambivalent form of perfectionism associated with high self-regard but low regard for others" (p. 7).

Given that there stand to be both benefits and costs to vicarious hope, it can be surmised that there might be an optimal level of such hope to strive toward. Bovens (1999) suggests that hope follows Aristotle's principle of the mean, wherein a moderate amount of a character trait is most adaptive; above and below this magnitude, maladaptive aspects of the trait will manifest. Bovens identifies *despair* as representing an unfavourably low amount of hope and *presumption* an unfavourably high amount of hope. This form of analysis may apply equally well to other-oriented hope. Indeed, Beste (2005) speaks of *fostering* the hope of others rather than instilling or controlling the hope of others. Fostering may be viewed as the Aristotlian mean between having no other-oriented hope and striving to instill or control it with too much fervor. In another analysis of the optimum level of hope, McGeer (2004) argues for *responsive hope* being an optimal point between wishful hope, on the one hand (i.e., desire but too little agency, as in *wishful thinking*) and willful hope, on the other hand (desire but too much agency, as in an incautious or unrealistic pursuit of one's dreams). To expand on McGeer's views, *responsive other-oriented hope* would fall between wishful other-oriented hope, on the one hand (i.e., desires aimed at others but divorced from an action-orientation toward the fulfillment of such desires), and willful other-oriented hope, on the other hand (i.e., desire for, and overzealous facilitation of, others' future outcomes, ignoring whether such actions are in the other's best interest or are endorsed by the other).

Salzberg (1995) gives the following example of the necessity of balancing our hope directed toward others and our ultimate need to accept that their fate is not under our control:

> We wish wholeheartedly, with great intensity, that they be free of suffering, that they be happy. But, in the end, we have to recognize where the boundaries actually are, what our responsibility really is, and where the source of happiness truly lies. If that friend does not change their behavior, they will suffer no matter how long and ardently we wish otherwise. (p. 147)

Finally, it bears recognizing that vicarious hope may at times take on a malevolent rather than a benevolent form, such as in the case of hoping that an ill-fate befalls another. In some cases, malevolent other-oriented hope would overlap with hatred, defined as "a motive associated with the goal of destroying or diminishing the object's well-being" (Rempel and Burris 2005, p. 300). Malevolent other-oriented hope, accompanied or not accompanied by hateful feelings, would have the impact of undermining another person's future, perhaps in order to enhance one's own good fortune or as a vengeful act to right perceived wrongs. Certain contexts may predict the occurrence of such malevolent other-oriented hope, including competitive or *zero-sum* situations in which one perceives that the other's gain is one's own loss. Personality predictors of malevolent hope would presumably include low agreeableness and more extreme traits such as psychopathy or narcissism. Consequences of such non-supportive or detrimental hope toward others would include erosion of the relationship, undermining of performance for the target of such hope and, at least in some cases, feelings of guilt or shame for the bearer of such hope.

However, some have argued that an intrinsic aspect of hope is that it concerns outcomes that can be seen as objectively good; for example, Averill et al. (1990) argue for a *rule of hope* in which hope concerns only socially acceptable ends. Similarly, Nunn (2005) argued that true hope is morally good, that is, that it takes into account the interests of others (see also Chap. 7). And, our view of vicarious hope as comprising one element of *other-interest* (see below) means that other-oriented hope, by necessity, concerns desirable outcomes for another person, that is, outcomes in that other person's best interest. Adopting such a view of other-oriented hope thereby precludes the possibility of hateful hope directed toward others, without denying that hateful impulses, acts, desires, or thoughts toward others nevertheless can and do occur.

## 5.4 Theoretical Frameworks for Understanding Other-Oriented Hope

In this section, we examine theoretical frameworks that can facilitate our understanding of vicarious hope. None of these frameworks have directly considered other-oriented hope, but they nonetheless are pertinent to understanding its nature and occurrence.

### *5.4.1 Other-Oriented Hope as a Manifestation of Other-Interest*

One framework for considering other-oriented hope is that of Gerbasi and Prentice's (2013) conceptualization of other-interest. As introduced in Chap. 2, this perspective argues that people have and invest interest in pursuits that forward their own gains, the gains of others, or the gains of both themselves and others. Within this perspective, self- and other-interest are viewed as two separable motivational dimensions underlying behaviour; as such, they are not necessarily antithetical or opposing, in that an individual may show high self- and other-interest simultaneously (or low self- and other-interest, or a high degree of one and a low degree of the other). According to Gerbasi and Prentice, other-interest may be fueled by human interdependence, such that behaviours expressive of other-interest may ultimately benefit the self. They further state that other-interest may reflect altruistic proclivities, such as high degrees of trait empathy or momentarily heightened state empathy.

Other-oriented hope may be a specific subtype of other-interest. Indeed, in the next chapter, we argue that other-interest encapsulates several interrelated concepts including other-oriented hope, compassion, altruism, empathy, caring, and love. As a subtype of other-interest, and as a form of hope, other-oriented hope reflects unique features of future-orientation, low certainty, and low controllability over outcomes. Moreover, other-oriented hope, like other-interest more generally, may be motivated by the interdependence characterizing our relationships with others, such as in the case of hope directed toward family members who, in turn, may be more likely to be available to provide similar support in a reciprocal manner in the future. Also, like other-interest more generally, other-oriented hope may be motivated by stable empathic dispositions or temporary empathic emotional states, such as in the case of hope toward an ill child by parents whose compassion is deeply invoked in response to such vulnerability. And, just as other-interest is said to reflect that humans' lives are richly socially embedded (Brewer 2004), other-oriented hope suggests the deeply social nature of hope, not only in that our hope is often influenced by, and concerns, those around us, but that our parents or other caregivers are initially "keepers of our hope until we are enabled, by their hope in us, to become agents of hope in our own right" (McGeer 2004, p. 108).

Therefore, other-oriented hope can be seen as one manifestation of the broader concept of other-interest. It is, in this view, one means by which we experience, and can express, our broader and more encompassing interest and investment in others' well-being.

### *5.4.2 Other-Oriented Hope as a Reflection of Self-Transcendence*

A second perspective germane to understanding other-oriented hope is Reed's (2008) theory of self-transcendence. Other-oriented hope may be viewed as a reflection of self-transcendence, a process often initiated in response to challenging life circumstances. Working within a nursing context, Reed defines self-transcendence as "the capacity to expand self-boundaries intrapersonally… interpersonally…temporally… and transpersonally" (p. 107). Reed argues that self-transcendence is a psychological process invoked by experiences of vulnerability (e.g., threatening health events) which often leads, somewhat paradoxically, to enhanced well-being. In congruence with Reed's theory, Coward (1996) showed that self-transcendence, as measured with the Self-Transcendence Scale, correlated significantly with both hope and well-being. Reed's model is compatible with arguments by Lazarus (1991) that hope (and, very possibly other-oriented hope) is typically a response to negative, challenging situations in which the person is "fearing the worst but yearning for better" (p. 282).

Tornstam (2011) also writes of the importance of transcendence, highlighting the potential relevance of transcendence to other-oriented hope. Based upon numerous qualitative and quantitative studies, Tornstam argues that *gerotranscendence* is characterized by existential changes such as a closer connection to earlier generations, changes to self-related processes such as reduced self-centeredness, and changes in relationships such as increased importance of close friendships and reduced materialism. Tornstam provides evidence that transcendence increases with age, is positively associated with life satisfaction, and is often triggered by life crises. Emphasizing the other-oriented nature of gerotranscendence, Tornstam states:

> Looking back, the individual notices how the focus on one's own needs has gradually been transcended and replaced with a focus on the needs of others – in particular the needs of children and grandchildren. Egoism has been overshadowed by altruism. (p. 172)

Supporting the positive attributes characterizing self-transcendence, research with the Adult Self-Transcendence Inventory shows that transcendence is distinguishable from self-alienation experiences, that transcendence is associated with positive personality traits (e.g., conscientiousness, agreeableness, and emotional stability), and that transcendence is higher among those who engage in meditation practice (Levenson et al. 2005).

The self-transcendent nature of vicarious hope was seen in the work of Herth (1990, 1993) and Duggleby and colleagues (Duggleby and Wright 2005; Duggleby et al. 2012), who documented a pattern of increasing other-oriented hope among individuals with terminal or otherwise incapacitating illnesses. It is possible that such hope serves a coping function for those for whom self-oriented hope is in diminished supply. Barilan (2012) also describes the redirecting of patients' hope "beyond the embodied person" (p. 168) and toward the welfare of family members as a potentially adaptive means of addressing hope in the face of death. Barilan states, "...many people regard the good of their dear ones and their life projects as more valuable than their own physical well-being" (p. 168). Barilan further argues that hope often involves transcending suffering and death in the service of *promotion-focus goals* (i.e., growth-oriented ends deemed valuable by the individual). To direct one's hope toward others as one nears the end of one's life can be viewed as a growth-oriented and self-transcendent experience which, according to the framework of Reed (2008), will be associated with improved levels of psychological functioning as it reflects an adaptive acceptance of the reality of one's situation. Turning to the hope of one's spouse or of one's children as one approaches death may be a means by which one can continue to exert a positive influence and impact when other means for doing so are increasingly restricted.

Reed (2008) further argues that the process of self-transcendence can be triggered among nurses and other caregivers in response to another's vulnerability.

Evidence reviewed in Chap. 4 concerning the occurrence of vicarious hope among such caregivers is, therefore, consistent with Reed's self-transcendence model.

More generally, the self-transcending investment in others through other-oriented hope may be one means by which adults experience a sense of ongoing *generativity*, as per Erikson's (1974) theory of psychosocial development. Erikson defines generativity as "... the establishment, the guidance, and the enrichment of the living generation and the world it inherits" (p. 123). According to Erikson, the key virtue arising from this stage of life is *care*. In discussing this stage of adult development, Slater (2003) argues that establishing a sense of trust in childhood later allows the adults' interests to be inclusive of others' interests, the expression of which is especially played out in the role of parenting: "Parents extend their own boundaries to include their hopes and expectations for the child" (p. 59).

McAdams (2013) reviews a vast amount of quantitative and qualitative research concerning generativity, outlining several key features of it: generativity occurs in response both to a cultural demand for investment in later generations and an inner desire to do so; it reflects caring about others, 'believing in the species', committing to others, and taking actions aimed at supporting others; and it culminates in the composition of a narrative identity that provides meaning and purpose to one's life. McAdams shows that many forms of generativity peak in midlife, and that generativity is positively associated with mental health and flourishing. Finally, McAdams argues that *redemption* is often at the core of generativity; that is, adults view generativity as a way of arising above past limitations, challenges, ailments, and personal shortcomings.

Although the concept of generativity is often deemed relevant only to those who have reached midlife, Leffel (2008) emphasizes its relevance across a broader developmental range, including young adulthood. For example, Hinds (1988) argues that the fact that adolescents with cancer exhibit other-oriented hope, whereas healthy adolescents or those with substance abuse do not, suggests a greater maturation of the former group, such that they demonstrated a desire for generativity seen typically only among older adults.

Other-oriented hope can, therefore, be construed as a specific form of self-transcendence, in which future-oriented concerns regarding the self are downplayed relative to concerns for another, often in response to perceived vulnerability of the self or of the other.

**Box 5.2: Adolescence and Other-Oriented Hope**

Interested in learning more about adolescent experiences of hope and how we might work effectively with youth, Rachel King, a doctoral student who I (D. L.) supervise, recently completed her master's thesis in which she conducted a Basic Interpretive Inquiry (Merriam 2002) into adolescent girls' experiences of hope (King 2014). Using photographs representing hope taken by the four research participants, Ms. King interviewed the girls about their experiences. Contrary to long-standing conceptions of the self-involved adolescent (e.g., Elkind 1967), all four girls offered unsolicited dialogue about their other-oriented hopes. Other-oriented hopes were largely held for important others and included remarks like, "I always hope for the better for my siblings" (from a girl not currently in contact with her siblings), and "hoping for friends to no longer be bullied, hoping for parents to no longer have financial distress, and hoping for ex-boyfriends to be happy and move on" (p. 77). To represent her hope, one girl had taken a photo of a *pink-shirt day* anti-bullying poster in her school. Interestingly, another participant noted that it was often easier to hold hope for others than for herself, saying "I mostly hope for other people. I don't really hope for myself that much because when I hope for myself the things I hope for don't really happen so I mostly just hope for other people, for their lives to get better and stuff" (p. 77).

### *5.4.3 Other-Oriented Hope and Mental Balance*

A third framework within which to understand other-oriented hope arises from the consideration of Eastern perspectives on the understanding of optimal human functioning and well-being. Wallace and Shapiro (2006) present a fourfold model of mental health derived from the venerable psychological and philosophical framework of Buddhism. The model posits that mental health arises as a function of the achievement of balance in the domains of conation (motivation), attention, cognition, and emotion. A loss of balance in a domain will be expressed as deficits, excesses, or disturbances within that particular psychological function. The first and fourth domains (i.e., motivation and emotion) are most pertinent to the current focus.

With respect to motivational balance, Wallace and Shapiro (2006) argue that mental well-being is attained to the extent that one's desires and aspirations are appropriately directed toward *both* one's own and others' happiness. They identify wholesome goals and desires as those that facilitate one's own and others' well-being. Deficits in this domain involve hopelessness for one's own and others' futures, and excesses in this domain involve rigid fixation on one's own goals and neglect of the goals of others. Finally, dysfunction in this domain involves desiring things detrimental to one's own or others' well-being, or being indifferent to those things that do enhance well-being for oneself or others. Wallace and Shapiro state that:

> It is crucial to recognize that individual psychological flourishing is not something that can be cultivated while ignoring the well-being of others. People do not exist independently from others, so their well-being cannot arise independently of others either. (p. 694)

Wallace and Shapiro (2006) further argue that conative balance is required before balance can be attained in the attentional, cognitive, and affective domains. Finally, the cultivation of *right motivation* (i.e., an appropriate balance within the conative domain) occurs through meditative practices, which include "reflection on meaningful and wholesome desires and recognizing unwholesome desires that will lead to suffering both for oneself and others" (p. 694).

A second domain of balanced mental functioning pertinent to other-oriented hope is affective balance, which involves emotional stability and freedom from emotional apathy and inappropriate emotions. A deficit in this domain is manifested in emotional coldness, including "cold indifference toward others" (Wallace and Shapiro 2006, p. 698). Hyperactivity in this domain involves extremes of emotional experience, such as excess hope (presumably including excess other-oriented hope) and excess fear, excess adulation and excess contempt. Finally, dysfunction in this domain manifests as emotions inappropriate to the context, such as experiencing joy in relation to another's failure (i.e., *Schadenfreude*). Importantly, affective imbalances can be countered with meditation practices aimed at cultivating the states of consciousness of loving-kindness, compassion, empathic joy, and equanimity (Wallace and Shapiro 2006). Kindness and compassion are straightforwardly relevant to other-oriented hope. Although empathic joy chiefly arises upon contemplating another's current success, in the event that the thought-of individual is not currently in a joyful state it is advised that the target person's future good-fortune should be contemplated, thereby resembling other-oriented hope. For example, meditation to cultivate empathic joy includes a variation applicable to occasions when the individual at the focus of the contemplation is not currently experiencing a joyous state. The meditator is advised to contemplate that, "In the future he will again enjoy similar success and will go about in gold palanquins, on the backs of elephants or on horseback, and so on" (p. 308; Buddhaghosa 1995). Finally, equanimity is defined as "an impartial sense of caring for others' well-being, regardless of one's own self-centered likes and dislikes" (Wallace and Shapiro 2006, p. 698). Such an affective state would be conducive to the regular occurrence of other-oriented hope.

The developmental psychologist and empathy researcher Nancy Eisenberg (2002) also discusses the merits of cultivating kindness, compassion, empathic joy, and equanimity, stating "Buddhists have thought a lot about the importance of being other-oriented toward all individuals and of ways to counteract our tendencies to become prey to emotions such as envy, hostility, anxiety, and frustration that can undermine prosocial efforts" (p. 133). Other-oriented hope can be understood within this framework, given its emphasis on the importance for well-being of maintaining an inclusive orientation toward others.

### *5.4.4 Other-Oriented Hope and the Ecosystem Motivational Perspective*

A fourth and final perspective for understanding vicarious hope is the *egosystem versus ecosystem* motivational perspective. According to Crocker and colleagues (Crocker 2008; Crocker and Canevello 2008, 2012; Crocker et al. 2009), goals concerning one's interpersonal relationships can primarily take one of two forms. First, *self-image goals* emphasize the importance of establishing oneself as a competent, capable individual. Self-report questionnaire items employed to measure the self-image goals orientation include *avoid the possibility of being wrong, convince others that you are right,* and *get others to recognize or acknowledge your positive qualities*. Self-image goals are associated with what Crocker and colleagues refer to as an *egosystem* motivational perspective, in which one's own needs are placed above those of others, and relationships with others are construed as competitive, or zero-sum.

Second, *compassionate goals* emphasize the importance of being a caring, empathic, and considerate individual. Self-report questionnaire items employed to measure the compassionate goals orientation include *be constructive in your comments to others, avoid doing anything that would be harmful to others*, and *be supportive of others*. Compassionate goals are associated with what Crocker et al. (2009) refer to as an *ecosystem* motivational perspective, in which an emphasis is placed upon caring about and being responsive to the needs and well-being of others, and relationships with others are construed as potentially mutually beneficial, or non-zero-sum. Importantly, there is evidence that the adoption of compassionate goals relative to self-image goals is conducive to well-being (Crocker et al. 2009).

To experience and express other-oriented hope is congruent with the adoption of compassionate goals and an ecosystem motivational perspective. People who aim to be considerate and caring toward others are more likely to harbour hopes for others relative to those who aim to establish themselves as competent and capable individuals. Indeed, it may be the case that adoption of the ecosystem perspective promotes other-oriented hope, whereas adoption of an egosystem perspective promotes self-oriented hope.

These four theoretical perspectives pertinent to vicarious hope (i.e., other-interest, self-transcendence, mental balance, and the ecosystem motivational orientation) share several commonalities with each other and with other-oriented hope. First, they all emphasize the importance of our relationships with others and, as a result, our willingness to take into account others' interests. Second, they all argue that the inclusion of others in our scope of interest may have benefits for our own psychological health and adaptive functioning. Third, these perspectives, taken together, allow that our interest in others is, to a degree, traded-off with (and hence requires balance with) our self-interest. Finally, these perspectives are each congruent with arguments that positive psychological functioning often reflects a reduced self-focus. Indeed, heightened well-being associated with a reduced self-focus has been described as occurring in several manifestations, including in the form of ego-quieting (Bauer 2008), hypoegoic functioning (Leary et al. 2006; Leary and Guadagno 2011), or self-environment harmony (Dambrun and Ricard 2011). According to Bauer (2008), for example, well-being requires balancing self- and other-interest via a quieting of the ego, therefore promoting characteristics such as gratitude, compassion, and humility.

In addition to these similarities, there are unique aspects of these perspectives vis a vis their relationship with other-oriented hope. First, the self-transcendence perspective (and to a lesser degree the mental balance perspective) gives a prominent role to feelings of vulnerability in initiating a shift toward greater concern with others. This can be seen as a key point, given evidence reviewed in Chap. 4 that other-oriented hope frequently occurs under conditions of one's own or others' vulnerability. Second, each of the perspectives describes personal traits and momentary states that may be conducive to other-oriented hope, such as an altruistic personality, states of compassion and lovingkindness, experiences of transcendence, and the adoption of compassionate goals. Third, only the mental balance perspective provides a direct route to enhance one's mental functioning to more fully take into account the needs of others, through specific meditation practices. Finally, the other-interest and ecosystem perspectives are distinctive in that each of them contrasts an aspect of our functioning that is other-oriented (i.e., other-interest and compassionate goals, respectively) with an aspect of our functioning that is self-oriented (i.e., self-interest and self-image goals, respectively). This, of course, is similar to the contrast between other-oriented hope and self-oriented hope.

In the following chapter, we examine the similarity and distinctiveness of other-oriented hope in comparison to numerous related concepts, such as love and caring.

## References


Aronson, E., & Patnoe, S. (1997). *The jigsaw classroom: Building cooperation in the classroom* (2nd ed.). New York: Addison Wesley Longman.

Averill, J. R., Catlin, G., & Chon, K. K. (1990). *Rules of hope*. New York: Springer.

Bailie, T. (2014). *Effects of compassion on vicarious hope and vicarious gratitude*. Unpublished honour's thesis.

Barilan, Y. M. (2012). From hope in palliative care to hope as a virtue and a life skill. *Philosophy, Psychiatry, and Psychology, 19*, 165–181.

Batson, C. D., & Shaw, L. L. (1991). Evidence for altruism: Toward a pluralism of prosocial motives. *Psychological Inquiry, 2*, 107–122.

Bauer, J. J. (2008). How the ego quiets as it grows: Ego development, growth stories, and eudaimonic personality development. In H. A. Wayment & J. J. Bauer (Eds.), *Transcending self-interest: Psychological explorations of the quiet ego* (pp. 199–209). Washington, DC: American Psychological Association.

Beste, J. (2005). Instilling hope and respecting patient autonomy: Reconciling apparently conflicting duties. *Bioethics, 19*, 215–231.

Bovens, L. (1999). The value of hope. *Philosophy and Phenomenological Research, 59*, 667–681.

Brewer, M. B. (2004). Taking the social origins of human nature seriously: Toward a more imperialist social psychology. *Personality and Social Psychology Review, 8*, 107–113.

Buddhaghosa, B. (1995). *The path of purification*. Seattle, WA: Buddhist Publication Society.

Cherrington, A. (2013). *Exploring hope from the perspective of South African children made vulnerable due to HIV & AIDS: An arts-based approach*. Unpublished manuscript. Nelson Mandela Metro University, Port Elizabeth, South Africa.

Coward, D. (1996). Self-transcendence and correlates in a healthy population. *Nursing Research, 45*, 116–122.

Crocker, J. (2008). From egosystem to ecosystem: Implications for learning, relationships, and well-being. In H. Wayment & J. Brauer (Eds.), *Transcending self-interest: Psychological explorations of the quiet ego* (pp. 63–72). Washington, DC: American Psychological Association.

Crocker, J., & Canevello, A. (2008). Creating and undermining social support in communal relationships: The role of compassionate and self-image goals. *Journal of Personality and Social Psychology, 95*, 555–575.

Crocker, J., & Canevello, A. (2012). Consequences of self-image and compassionate goals. *Advances in Experimental Social Psychology, 45*, 229–278.

Crocker, J., Olivier, M. A., & Nuer, N. (2009). Self-image goals and compassionate goals: Costs and benefits. *Self Identity, 8*, 251–269.

Dambrun, M., & Ricard, M. (2011). Self-centeredness and selflessness: A theory of self-based psychological functioning and its consequences for happiness. *Review of General Psychology, 15*, 138–157.

Day, J. P. (1969). Hope. *American Philosophical Quarterly, 6*, 89–102.

Duggleby, W., Hicks, D., Nekolaichuk, C., Holtslander, L., Williams, A., Chambers, T., & Eby, J. (2012). Hope, older adults, and chronic illness: A metasynthesis of qualitative research. *Journal of Advanced Nursing, 68*, 1211–1223.

Duggleby, W., & Wright, K. (2005). Transforming hope: How elderly palliative patients live with hope. *Canadian Journal of Nursing Research, 37*, 70–84.

Eisenberg, N. (2002). Empathy-related emotional responses, altruism, and their socialization. In R. J. Davidson & A. Harrington (Eds.), *Visions of compassion: Western scientists and Tibetan Buddhists examine human nature* (pp. 131–164). New York: Oxford University Press.

Eisenberg, N., & Lennon, R. (1983). Sex differences in empathy and related capacities. *Psychological Bulletin, 94*, 100–131.

Eliott, J. A., & Olver, I. N. (2007). Hope and hoping in the talk of dying cancer patients. *Social Science and Medicine, 64*, 138–149.

Elkind, D. (1967). Egocentrism in adolescence. *Child Development, 38*, 1025–1034.

Erikson, E. H. (1974). *Dimensions of a new identity*. New York: Norton.

Faso, D. J., Neal-Beevers, A. R., & Carlson, C. L. (2013). Vicarious futurity, hope, and well-being in parents of children with autism spectrum disorder. *Research in Autism Spectrum Disorders, 7*, 288–297.

Gable, S. L., Gonzaga, G. C., & Strachman, A. (2006). Will you be there for me when things go right? Supportive responses to positive event disclosures. *Journal of Personality and Social Psychology, 91*, 904–917.

Gable, S. L., & Reis, H. T. (2010). Good news! Capitalizing on positive events in an interpersonal context. *Advances in Experimental Social Psychology, 42*, 195–257.

Gable, S. L., Reis, H. T., Impett, E. A., & Asher, E. R. (2004). What do you do when things go right? The intrapersonal and interpersonal benefits of sharing positive events. *Journal of Personality and Social Psychology, 87*, 228–245.

Gerbasi, M. E., & Prentice, D. A. (2013). The Self- and Other-Interest Inventory. *Journal of Personality and Social Psychology, 105*, 495–514.

Harvey, J. H., Pauwels, B. G., & Zickmund, S. (2002). Relationship connection: The role of minding in enhancement of closeness. In C. R. Snyder & S. J. Lopez (Eds.), *Handbook of positive psychology* (pp. 423–433). New York: Oxford University Press.

Hernandez, M., Barrio, C., & Yamada, A.-M. (2013). Hope and burden among Latino families of adults with schizophrenia. *Family Process, 52*, 697–708.

Herth, K. (1990). Fostering hope in terminally-ill people. *Journal of Advanced Nursing, 13*, 1250–1259.

Herth, K. (1993). Hope in older adults in community and institutional settings. *Issues in Mental Health Nursing, 14*, 139–156.

Hewitt, P. L., & Flett, G. L. (2004). *Multidimensional Perfectionism Scale (MPS): Technical manual*. Toronto: Multi-Health Systems.

Hinds, P. S. (1988). Adolescent hopefulness in illness and health. *Advances in Nursing Science, 10*, 79–88.

Hollis, V., Massey, K., & Jevne, R. (2007). An introduction to the intentional use of hope. *Journal of Allied Health, 36*, 52–56.

Howell, A. J., Bailie, T., & Buro, K. (in press). Evidence for vicarious hope and vicarious gratitude. *Journal of Happiness Studies.*

King, R. (2014). *Small laughs: Understanding hope in early adolescent girls.* Unpublished Master's thesis. University of Alberta, Edmonton, Alberta, Canada.

Kopelowicz, A., Zarate, R., Gonzalez Smith, V., Mintz, J., & Liberman, R. P. (2003). Disease management in Latinos with schizophrenia: A family-assisted, skills training approach. *Schizophrenia Bulletin, 29*, 211–227.

Langston, C. A. (1994). Capitalizing on and coping with daily-life events: Expressive responses to positive events. *Journal of Personality and Social Psychology, 67*, 132–140.

Larsen, D. J., Stege, R., & Flesaker, K. (2013). 'It's important for me not to let go of hope': Psychologists' in-session experiences of hope. *Reflective Practice: International and Multidisciplinary Perspectives, 14*, 472–486.

Lazarus, R. S. (1991). *Emotion and adaptation.* New York: Oxford University Press.

Lazarus, R. S. (1999). Hope: An emotion and a vital coping resource against despair. *Social Research, 66*, 653–678.

Leary, M. R., Adams, C. E., & Tate, E. B. (2006). Hypo-egoic self-regulation: Exercising self-control by diminishing the influence of the self. *Journal of Personality, 74*, 1803–1831.

Leary, M. R., & Guadagno, J. (2011). The role of hypo-egoic self-processes in optimal functioning and subjective well-being. In K. M. Sheldon, T. B. Kashdan, & M. F. Steger (Eds.), *Designing positive psychology: Taking stock and moving forward* (pp. 135–146). New York: Oxford University Press.

Leffel, G. M. (2008). Who cares? Generativity and the moral emotions, Part 2: A "social intuitionist model" of moral motivation. *Journal of Psychology and Theology, 36*, 182–201.

Levenson, M. R., Jennings, P. A., Aldwin, C. M., & Shiraishi, R. W. (2005). Self-transcendence: Conceptualization and measurement. *International Journal of Aging and Human Development, 60*, 127–143.

Li, Y., & Larsen, D. J. (2012). Finding hope in the darkness: Stories of two Chinese newcomers enrolled in a Canadian high school. *Canadian and International Education, 41*, 39–58.

Mattos, A. (2009). *Narratives on teaching and teacher education: An international perspective.* New York: Palgrave MacMillan.

McAdams, D. P. (2013). The positive psychology of adult generativity: Caring for the next generation and constructing a redemptive life. In J. D. Sinnott (Ed.), *Positive Psychology: Advances in Understanding Adult Motivation* (pp. 191–205). New York: Springer.

McGeer, V. (2004). The art of good hope. *Annals of the American Academy of Political and Social Science, 592*, 100–127.

Merriam, S. B. (2002). *Introduction to qualitative research.* San Francisco: Jossey-Bass.

Nunn, B. V. (2005). Getting clear what hope is. In J. A. Eliott (Ed.), *Interdisciplinary perspectives on hope* (pp. 63–77). New York: Nova Science Publishers.

Reed, P. (2008). Theory of self-transcendence. In M. J. Smith & P. Liehr (Eds.), *Middle range theory for nursing* (pp. 105–129). New York: Springer.

Rempel, J. K., & Burris, C. T. (2005). Let me count the ways: An integrative theory of love and hate. *Personal Relationships, 12*, 297–313.

Salzburg, S. (1995). *Lovingkindness: The revolutionary art of happiness.* Boston: Shambhala Publications.

Simpson, C. (2004). When hope makes us vulnerable: A discussion of patient-healthcare provider interactions in the context of hope. *Bioethics, 18*, 428–447.

Slater, C. L. (2003). Generativity versus stagnation: An elaboration of Erikson's adult stage of human development. *Journal of Adult Development, 10*, 53–65.

Snyder, C. R. (2002). Hope theory: Rainbows in the mind. *Psychological Inquiry, 13*, 1047–1084.

Stoeber, J. (2014). How other-oriented perfectionism differs from self-oriented and socially prescribed perfectionism. *Journal of Psychopathology and Behavioral Assessment, 40*, 329–338.

Tornstam, L. (2011). Maturing into gerotranscendence. *Journal of Transpersonal Psychology, 43*, 166–180.

Triandis, H. C., Bontempo, R., & Villareal, M. J. (1988). Individualism and collectivism: Cross-cultural perspectives on self-ingroup relationships. *Journal of Personality and Social Psychology, 54*, 323–338.

Van Lange, P. A. M., Bekkers, R., Schuyt, T. N. M., & Van Vugt, M. (2007). From games to giving: Social value orientation predicts donations to noble causes. *Basic and Applied Social Psychology, 29*, 375–384.

van Manen, M. (2002). Care-as-worry, or Don't worry, be happy. *Qualitative Health Research, 12*, 262–278.

Wallace, B. A., & Shapiro, S. L. (2006). Mental balance and well-being: Building bridges between Buddhism and Western psychology. *American Psychologist, 61*, 690–701.

Weingarten, K. (2010). Reasonable hope: Construct, clinical applications, and supports. *Family Process, 49*, 5–25.

Wong, M. G., & Heriot, S. A. (2008). Parents of children with cystic fibrosis: How they hope, cope, and despair. *Child: Care, Health and Development, 34*, 344–354.

# Chapter 6
# Other-Oriented Hope and Related Concepts

## 6.1 General

*...Hope and certain forms of care have much in common...*
—Barilan 2012, p. 167

*Hoping and fearing for the well-being of a loved one are constitutive of loving.*
—Bovens 1999, p. 676

Other-oriented hope is likely to fall within a nomological network of overlapping but differentiable concepts. In our view, that network of associated concepts is hierarchically organized, with the superordinate concept being that of *other-interest*. Subordinate concepts, each reflecting a manner in which other-interest comes to be enacted, include other-oriented hope, altruism, compassion, empathy, love, caring, and worry. In this penultimate chapter, we examine the commonalities and distinctions among other-oriented hope and each of these related concepts.

## 6.2 Other-Oriented Hope and Other-Interest

As outlined in Chaps. 2 and 5, other-interest describes an overall motivational orientation toward looking out for the welfare of others, reflecting a desire to help and support others and valuing and celebrating others' well-being (Gerbasi and Prentice 2013). According to Gerbasi and Prentice, being motivated to help others may reflect one's interdependence on others (i.e., other-interest can be a means to other ends) or one's inherent concern toward those others (i.e., other-interest can be an end in and of itself). Other-interest is contrasted by Gerbasi and Prentice with self-interest, which describes an overall motivational orientation toward looking out for one's own welfare. Furthermore, Gerbasi and Prentice argue that many behaviours are motivated by a mix of other- and self-interest working in tandem with each other.



A.J. Howell and D.J. Larsen, *Understanding Other-Oriented Hope*,
SpringerBriefs in Well-Being and Quality of Life Research,
DOI 10.1007/978-3-319-15007-9_6

Other-oriented hope can be seen as a specific component of the broader concept of other-interest. Indeed, we view other-interest as a superordinate concept, within which falls other-oriented hope. Other-oriented hope and other-interest both involve an orientation to the other, that is, a willingness to place importance on the interests and welfare of another person. Both have alternative and contrasting forms (i.e., *self*-interest and *self*-oriented hope), allowing for the differentiation of hope or interest that is applied to others versus hope or interest that is applied to the self. Both affect how we behave with respect to others, in that other-oriented hope and other-interest lead us to take steps toward the attainment, recognition, or maintenance of desired outcomes for the other. Finally, both are viewed as occurring in tandem with, rather than in opposition to, their self-focused counterparts; that is, other-oriented hope and other-interest are not seen as antithetical to self-oriented hope and self-interest, respectively, but rather are viewed as separable, but often co-occurring, influences on how we think and behave. Just as one can simultaneously experience self- and other-interest, and one's current behaviour can reflect both influences, one can also have concurrent hopes for oneself and for others which may also simultaneously exert influence on our behaviour.

The overlap between domains of other-interest and other-oriented hope is revealed in the manner in which other-interest is operationalized by Gerbasi and Prentice (2013) in the form of their Self- and Other-Interest Inventory. On this measure, several items used to measure other-interest refer to a future-oriented, uncertain anticipation of good fortunes for others (e.g., *I am constantly looking for ways for my classmates to get ahead*; *I look for opportunities to help people I know achieve higher social status*); other items, however, are more neutral with respect to the time perspective inherent within them (e.g., *The success of my friends is important to me; It is important to me that others are happy*). Other-interest includes appreciating and supporting a person's past or present successes in addition to more future-oriented desires for others' well-being.

Thus, a main distinction between other-interest and other-oriented hope is the more restricted time perspective attached to the latter (i.e., generally a future orientation). Whereas other-interest concerns the past, present, and future well-being of another, the forward-looking nature of other-oriented hope brings the future time perspective into full relief. A corollary of this difference is that other-oriented hope is imbued with uncertainty and anticipation to a greater degree than is other-interest. Finally, because we view other-oriented hope as subsumed within the higher-order concept of other-interest, all instances of other-oriented hope will express other-interest, whereas not all instances of other-interest will express other-oriented hope. Other-oriented hope is the narrower concept, focused squarely upon future-oriented thinking surrounding desired but uncertain outcomes for others.

## 6.3 Other-Oriented Hope and Altruism

If other-oriented hope reflects other-interest, a related issue concerns the extent to which other-oriented hope can be viewed as being altruistic in nature. Indeed, instances of other-oriented hope have been termed *altruistic hope* (Averill et al. 1990; Bruininks and Malle 2005). The degree to which other-oriented hope can be construed as altruistic hope is a challenging issue, no less challenging than the attempt to establish any behaviour or mental process as rooted wholly in selfless motives.

Penner and Orom (2010) define altruistic behaviour as "... behaviour in which the sole motivation for the action is to improve another person's well-being, with there being no expectation of tangible or even intangible rewards" (p. 56). We make no claims that other-oriented hope is necessarily altruistic in nature. Recall that we define other-oriented hope as *future-oriented belief, desire, and mental imagining surrounding a valued outcome of another person that is uncertain but possible.* This definition describes the *act* of hoping for others, but not whether the *motivation* behind the hoping reflects only a concern regarding another's well-being. Correspondingly, none of the research described herein has definitively shown that instances of other-oriented hope reflect an altruistic motivation. Indeed, the vast majority of studies yielding evidence of other-oriented hope have been descriptive in nature. For example, studies reviewed in Chap. 4 showed that parents and other caregivers of loved ones who are ill often harbour other-oriented hope toward the loved one; it is impossible to discern from such observations the extent to which hope held for others is altruistic in nature. Nonetheless, the repeated finding of evidence consistent with the notion of other-oriented hope is a precondition for the existence of altruistic forms of hope; a repeated lack of evidence for other-oriented hope would falsify claims concerning the existence of altruistic hope.

Other-oriented hope can be viewed as an aspect of *prosocial behaviour*, defined by Penner and Orom (2010) as "... any act intended to benefit another person or entity; the motivation responsible for that act is not considered" (p. 56). When so viewed, other-oriented hope is not assumed strictly to be motivated by altruism. Indeed, forms of behaviour that are wholly altruistic may be few and far between. For example, hoping that a parent recovers from a serious illness can reflect genuine concern for the welfare of that parent, and nothing more. At the same time, it can reflect the desire to be freed from the responsibility of taking care of the parent. In this way, such hope reveals a blend of both altruistic and egoistic motivations.

This dualism can be seen in an actual clinical example. In her in-depth description of the case of a man whose partner was dying of AIDS-related dementia, Kelly (2007) reports that the man's hope came to include hoping for the partner's death. While this can be seen as hope that is in the patient's best interest (e.g., reducing unnecessary suffering if improvement in functioning cannot be attained), the man also stated, "Tom's going to be a millstone around my neck for the rest of my life" (Kelly 2007, p. 870). Though unrealistic in nature (i.e., the well partner will very likely outlive the ill partner), this concern also acknowledges the expected and necessary self-interest which is at stake when one is committed to caring for another: To care for another who is incapacitated by illness requires an often considerable degree of self-sacrifice, in which one's own needs are at least temporarily put on hold or considered secondary in importance. There are limits to such self-sacrifice, however; it cannot be absolute. As stated by Mansbridge (1990), "altruism must coincide with self-interest sufficiently to prevent the extinction of either the altruistic motive or the altruist" (p. 133). In a similar vein, Frimer et al. (2011) describe the integration and alignment of self- and other-concerns documented among a group of moral exemplars as *enlightened self-interest,* and argue that such a concept should replace the notion of altruism.

Even though other-oriented hope cannot unequivocally be established as altruistic hope, there are several reasons for making and valuing a distinction between other- and self-oriented hope. First, we view the distinction between other- and self-oriented hope as being as well-established as other ways in which types of hope have been differentiated from each other. Just as some instances of hope concern long-term outcomes whereas some focus upon more immediate concerns, just as some concern relatively certain outcomes and many concern uncertain outcomes, just as some concern extrinsic values and others concern intrinsic ones, just as some concern controllable outcomes whereas others concern uncontrollable ones, just as some are largely cognitive whereas other experiences are more emotional, just as some concern goals whereas others focus on process, instances of hope differ as to whether they focus upon the welfare of another or are baldly self-focused. While much hope will occupy a more ambiguous position between the two poles of self- and other-oriented, the same is true also with respect to the aforementioned dimensions along which hope can vary. The tendency to experience hope that falls to either side of these various distinctions, in our view, is worthy of ongoing research and theoretical consideration.

Second, it can be argued that other-oriented hope, regardless of its underlying motivation, is an important domain of hope and is worthy of empirical scrutiny. Just as some researchers are interested in prosocial behaviour regardless of its underlying motivation (Penner and Orom 2010), the study of other-oriented hope may yield important advances in our understanding of hope independent of whether other-oriented hope is viewed as necessarily reflecting altruistic motivation. For example, the dualism of hope focused on the self or on others has been included in various multidimensional conceptualizations of hope (e.g., Eliott and Olver 2002), without conflating this dimension with the issue of altruistic versus selfish hope. Therefore, empirical work on other-oriented hope can help to establish the degree to which hope does vary along this dimension, supporting or disconfirming models of hope which include such a distinction.

Third, while it could be asserted that perhaps no instance of hope is wholly altruistic, as even a seemingly selfless hope could be seen to have self-relevant undertones, it could as readily be asserted that no instance of hope is wholly self-concerned. So, just as other-oriented hope not taken at face value may be seen as disguising underlying selfish motives, a self-oriented hope not taken at face value may be seen as disguising underlying altruistic motives. For example, hoping to secure a well-paying job could reflect the desire to personally attain a position of wealth and status among one's peers. Or, it could reflect an underlying motivation to adequately shelter, feed, and clothe one's children. That we less frequently consider this latter situation relative to the former suggests an inherent tendency to view human behaviour as self-interested (Miller 1999). However, if both other-oriented hope and self-oriented hope are judged on the basis of their outward features, then a fairer assessment of the self- versus other-regarding nature of hope can be cast. Just as the surface features of an outward behaviour can be used to judge a behaviour as prosocial (e.g., jumping into a lake to help a person who is drowning vs. not jumping), the surface features of a spoken or written narrative can be used to judge hope as other-oriented.

Fourth, and related to the point immediately above, significant headway has been made in operationalizing the distinction between other-oriented and self-oriented hope: there is evidence of the reliable classification of hope as other-oriented (e.g., Howell et al., in press; Lapierre et al. 2001; Newton et al. 2014). Fifth, evidence of the consistent coding of other-oriented hope has facilitated research validating the concept of other-oriented hope; that is, work (reviewed in earlier chapters) has validated the nature of other-oriented hope by documenting its empirical association with characteristics logically associated with heightened degrees of other-interest. For example, Herth (1993) demonstrated that other-oriented hope is found more frequently among very elderly individuals experiencing high levels of disability, in keeping with the notion that hope comes increasingly to be directed toward others when one's own future, or the ability to shape it, is limited. Newton et al. (2014) showed that other-oriented hope correlated positively with perceptions of one's own generativity, a concept which is itself most often conceptualized as other-oriented in nature. Howell et al. (in press) showed that the personality trait of empathic concern, perceived to be a main contributor to altruistic motivation behind helping others (Batson 2011), correlates positively with the frequency with which hope is other-oriented. Howell et al. (in press) also showed that other-oriented hope increases in frequency when participants are primed to take others into account as they generate their list of hoped-for outcomes, relative to participants not primed in this manner. That heightened accessibility of the concept of *other* leads to greater other-oriented hope is consistent with the unique and distinct nature of other-oriented hope.

In unpublished research, Bailie (2014) examined whether the manipulation of the emotional state of compassion leads to an increased frequency of other-oriented hope, premised upon the idea that the other-regarding emotion of compassion encourages greater consideration of others' hope. Undergraduate participants listed things for which they were hopeful after they watched a neutral slide show or a slide show validated to induce compassion. Results revealed more other-oriented hope among those in the compassion condition compared to those in the neutral condition. This finding fits within the framework in which other-oriented hope is conceived of as being prosocial in nature and as distinct from self-oriented hope.

Future work examining the antecedents, consequences, and sequelae of other-oriented hope will add to its ongoing validation as a form of hope distinct from self-oriented hope, even if other-oriented hope cannot be equated with altruistic hope. Meanwhile, progress is occurring in related domains of research concerning different physiological systems behind self- and other-oriented behaviour, further validating such a distinction. Indeed, based upon their review of evidence supporting the existence of a biological substrate for caregiving motivation and behaviour, Brown et al. (2012) state, "The existence of such a system poses a challenge to dominant views in psychology and the behavioral sciences that rely on concepts such as rational self-interest or psychological hedonism to explain social behavior" (p. 84).

## 6.4 Other-Oriented Hope and Compassion

Compassion is "the feeling that arises in witnessing another's suffering and that motivates a subsequent desire to help" (Goetz et al. 2010, p. 351). As with other emotions, compassion is said to guide thought and action in relation to one's goals. Compassion is especially pertinent to goals that are interpersonal in nature, such as the goal of fairness or the goal of forwarding another person's well-being. According to Goetz et al., compassion toward another is experienced to the extent that the other's suffering is incompatible with the witnesses' goals. Overall, compassion is associated with a reduced concern with one's own needs, and increased concern for the other (Goetz et al. 2010); compassion can also involve identification with the sufferer (Cassell 2002) and selflessness (Dambrun and Ricard 2011). For example, Oveis et al. (2010) showed that people with high scores on a measure of trait compassion, and those induced to experience state compassion, judged themselves to be more similar to weak or disadvantaged others relative to less compassionate people.

These properties of compassion—interpersonal goal-orientation, reduced self-focus, identification with the other—reflect that compassion is a means of embodying other-interest; as a result, compassion has a sibling relationship with other-oriented hope. Both compassion and vicarious hope reveal investment in the welfare of others. Compassion differs from other-oriented hope in that the latter does not require the suffering of another. For example, one can hold vicarious hope for someone concerning a positive striving, such as ongoing success in an academic endeavor; compassion likely would not be present in such a situation. On the other hand, compassion is implicated in situations involving harm to another person, especially unjustified harm (Goetz et al. 2010). Note, however, that it is the case that many instances of other-oriented hope do occur in response to another's plight. As we saw in Chap. 4, instances of other-oriented hope occur in the context of illness, leading parents to hope for their child's improved health, therapists to hope for their clients' further growth, or caregivers to hope for their loved one's recovery. In this way, compassion and other-oriented hope are likely to co-occur. Indeed, it is possible that compassion in response to another's vulnerability is a significant trigger for subsequent other-oriented hope.

This latter point highlights a further manner in which compassion and other-oriented hope are differentiable: compassion is chiefly a present-oriented state, whereas other-oriented hope is chiefly a future-oriented state. We feel compassion when another's current plight leads us to want to alleviate the other's distress. Other-oriented hope, in contrast, is a phenomenon that reaches further into the future, extending beyond the confines of the current situation. For example, whereas we feel compassion in response to seeing an injured child, other-oriented hope is reflected in our ongoing desire for the child to thrive in the future, long after the current concern has been resolved. Finally, compassion spurs the compassionate into action, seeking change for those in perceived need (Weingarten 2010). Other-oriented hope does not necessarily involve this inherent 'call-to-action'. Indeed, the potential for direct ameliorative action may or may not exist. Consider the hopes we hold for others that may not be actionable ourselves.

Similar to compassion is the concept of *compassionate love*. Underwood (2009; see also Oman 2011) defines compassionate love as "giving of the self for the good of the other" (p. 4), and illustrates its measurement with items emphasizing caring for others (e.g., *I feel a selfless caring for others*) and accepting others despite their shortcomings (e.g., *I accept others even when they do things I think are wrong*). Like other-oriented hope, compassionate love involves understanding the needs of the other. Compassionate love is concerned both with alleviating the suffering of another and enhancing the well-being of the other. Moreover, compassionate love can be directed toward any others, including those with whom we have intimate relationships, but also including strangers and all of humanity. Although these characteristics of compassionate love resemble features of other-oriented hope, the latter is significantly more future-oriented, imbued with uncertainty, and less tied to perceptions of vulnerability in the other. Moreover, while compassionate love emphasizes affective closeness with others, other-oriented hope has as its chief emotional element the experience of positive anticipation of a desired outcome.

## 6.5 Other-Oriented Hope and Empathy

Empathy is commonly conceptualized as involving both the ability to take the perspective of another person who is in need, and feeling empathic concern toward that other (Batson 2011; Davis 1983; de Waal 2008). According to Batson (2011), this latter emotional component, empathic concern, is more central to the experience of empathy than the cognitive component, perspective-taking. Batson argues that empathy overlaps with several related states "that are more other-focused than self-focused, including feelings of sympathy, compassion, tenderness, and the like" (Batson 1991, p. 86). Furthermore, Batson identifies empathic concern as a key feature of altruistic behaviour toward others; that is, upon observing another in need, the experience of empathic concern leads many individuals to provide help, even at the risk of sacrificing their own well-being.

**Box 6.1: The Mask of Hope**
Regan Holt, a junior high school teacher, has made fascinating observations when working with her junior high school students on hope. As part of the hope-infused curriculum in her classroom, Ms. Holt had her students create hope masks. With the help of classmates, youths made masks specifically fitted to their own faces. The youths were then instructed to paint their masks both outside and inside. The outside of the masks illustrated what each child intended to portray to the outside world. The children described this as their 'face to the world', a combination of selective authenticity and impression management. The inside of the masks were used to illustrate their personal hopes. Still protected by the apparent ambiguity of pictorial representations, these images represented the deeply held hopes of each boy or girl.

Once completed, the set of class masks were put on display in a protected glass cabinet in the school's main corridor. Some masks faced outward while others displayed the child's inner hopes. Of the many hope-focused activities Ms. Holt has done with her classes, this one stands out for her. She was taken with the length of time adults and children alike stopped to view the masks—they took their time—seemingly curious, caring about, empathizing with and investing in the hopes of the children.

One way in which empathy differs from other-oriented hope is that empathy is seen as a feeling that is *automatically elicited* in response to being exposed to a person in need. Other-oriented hope is more intentional and volitional than is empathy, although we speculate that the seeds of other-oriented hope may oftentimes be sown in an empathic response to another's plight. Another distinction between empathy and other-oriented hope is that the latter can occur independently of the suffering of another. The suffering of another is not a precondition of other-oriented hope, whereas it is of empathic responses. As such, while vicarious hope can concern the alleviation of another's distress or suffering, it can also be aimed at the occurrence of positive outcomes for an individual who is otherwise functioning well.

de Waal (2008) presents evidence that non-human primates (e.g., chimpanzees and apes) exhibit empathic reactions, reflecting basic evolved mechanisms such as emotional contagion; the fact that such primates presumably do not experience future-oriented concern for conspecifics further demonstrates a differentiation between empathy and other-oriented hope. Mechanisms for intentional helping and long-term care-providing among humans build upon, and go beyond, the common emotional core shared with our evolutionary ancestors.

The concept of *positive empathy* is even more akin to other-oriented hope. This concept has received very limited attention within psychological science. Buddhist ideology identifies *empathic joy* (*mudita*) as one of four key states of consciousness (along with lovingkindness, compassion, and equanimity) that are the target of cultivation in meditation practice (e.g., Salzberg 1995; Wallace and Shapiro 2006).

Empathic joy involves delighting in the positive experiences of another. This notion resembles *happy-for* emotional reactions, defined by emotion theorists Ortony et al. (1988) as being "pleased about an event presumed to be desirable for someone else" (p. 93). In their research, Sallquist et al. (2009) define positive empathy as "an expression of happiness or joy that results from comprehending another person's positive emotional state or condition" (p. 223). These researchers elicited positive empathy among preschool children by exposing the children to another person receiving a gift. They showed that children's positive empathic response to this event was associated with social competence, suggesting an adaptive function of positive empathy. Perry et al. (2012) showed that empathic responses to another person's joy (elicited by reading sentences such as *John won a scholarship*) were weaker than responses to another person's distress but nonetheless employed overlapping neural networks.

Research on positive empathy, although in its infancy, supports the overlap between empathy and other-oriented hope; however, like traditional research on (negative) empathy, positive empathy research continues to emphasize the emotional nature of the empathic response, the present-oriented time perspective of empathy, and the reflexive, automatic (as opposed to intentional and volitional) quality to this form of other-interest. Interestingly, this latter means of differentiating other-oriented hope from empathic reactions to another's emotional experience has recently been called into question. Zaki and Mitchell (2013) make the argument that prosocial decision-making and behaviour, perhaps including other-oriented hope, has an automatic aspect to it despite typically being viewed as controlled and deliberate. That is, they argue that prosociality can reflect the activity of an intuitive, "hot", automatic cognitive system as opposed to a reflective, "cool", controlled system. One line of evidence for this argument cited by Zaki and Mitchell is that infants show preference for prosocial over antisocial others before the age of 12 months, a developmental period during which more controlled forms of cognition and behaviour have yet to be acquired. Zaki and Mitchell state, "In many cases, prosocial acts, instead of requiring control over selfish impulses, may represent a class of intuition in and of themselves" (p. 469). Like prosocial acts, it is possible that prosocial hope, that is, other-oriented hope, can at times be automatically elicited. If this is the case, then the distinction between positive empathy and other-oriented hope is lessened, in that both processes may share an element of automaticity or intuition. Nonetheless, empathy and other-oriented hope continue to differ with respect to their temporal orientation: While empathy is in response to events of another person that are taking place in the current moment, other-oriented hope is focused upon the future welfare of the other, often including outcomes at a great distance in time from the present.

## 6.6 Other-Oriented Hope and Love

Love and hope (along with faith) are viewed as separate but interconnected theological virtues, suggesting an overlap between love and hope and, quite possibly, between love and other-oriented hope. Indeed, Bovens (1999) argues for a close connection between other-oriented hope and love, suggesting that love has as one of its constituents hoping for the loved one. Yet, he further suggests that the two are not synonymous, giving the poignant example of a parent's continued love for, but oftentimes absence of ongoing hope for, a deceased child.

In their analysis of love, Hegi and Bergner (2010) show that *investment in the well-being of the other for his or her own sake* is an important and perhaps essential feature of various forms of love, and that such investment is reflected especially in acts of support in times of need, avoiding harm, and furthering the goals and interests of the other. Rempel and Burris (2005) similarly define love as "a motivational state in which the goal is to preserve and promote the well-being of the valued object" (p. 299). While Hegi and Bergner's (2010) conceptualization equates love with altruism (Bergner and Ramon 2013), Rempel and Burris (2005) allow that love can reflect both self- and other-interest.

Each of these perspectives on love includes an aspect of desire for the other that is growth-oriented (i.e., furthering another's interests; promoting another's well-being), therefore underscoring a significant overlap with other-oriented hope. Indeed, other-oriented hope may be a particular form of psychological activity which reflects one's love for another. However, while vicarious hope is most likely to occur within the types of loving relationships identified by Hegi and Bergner (2010), such as romantic love and companionate love, it can occur in the absence of any form of loving relationship. For example, hope toward others can be harboured merely as a result of comprehending their plight, as in the case of hoping that victims of a natural disaster receive the medical aid that they require. And, it is possible that hope directed toward one person can ultimately be in the aim of aiding a third party, such that the presence of love toward the initial target of one's hope is not required. For example, one could hope that a politician has success in an election, but the ultimate aim of the hope is those who will benefit from improved social programs endorsed by that public figure. In such a case, no love or affection toward the politician is required for other-oriented hope to occur.

A further distinction between love and other-oriented hope is that the former emphasizes the close bond of affection between the parties, whereas the latter emphasizes specific or generalized preferences for another's future outcomes, and the anticipation of those outcomes. Love is therefore more emotionally-laden than is other-oriented hope, whereas other-oriented hope is more cognitively-laden than is love. But, these differences are only relative, as both experiences involve emotional *and* cognitive elements.

## 6.7 Other-Oriented Hope and Care

Care is an additional concept that overlaps with other-oriented hope. From a phenomenological perspective, van Manen (2002) characterizes the caring of parents toward their children as *care-as-worry*, emphasizing the virtually never-abating experience of parental worry regarding the well-being of their children (further discussion of hope and worry appears in the following section). While van Manen emphasizes the negatively-valenced future-oriented thinking that accompanies parental caring, care can involve looking ahead to positive possibilities as well; in this case, the overlap with other-oriented hope is increased. This is exemplified in van Manen's quotation from the diary of Judith Minty (1982): "It is much later now. He is sleeping. Everyone is sleeping. I hope his spirit sleeps well" (p. 217). Barilan (2012) more formally distinguishes between the focus upon alleviation of distress in care and the growth-oriented focus of hope.

From a psychological perspective, Hall (1990) characterizes the components of care as consisting of care beliefs or philosophies, care goals or objectives, care practices and acts, and care emotions and feelings. The first component bears little resemblance to other-oriented hope. While the second component of care goals and objectives would suggest compatibility with the concept of other-oriented hope, Hall argues that the goals of caring may be those which benefit the carer or which strive to attain externally defined objectives (e.g., related to care policy); in this way, the goals of caring are not necessarily other-oriented or reflective of high degrees of other-interest. The act of caring, as a third key component, is described as involving physical presence, aid with daily living activities and, often, physical contact; none of these aspects of caring require other-oriented hope or are necessary aspects of other-oriented hope. The fourth component concerning feelings and emotions are described by Hall as most typically involving negative feelings in relation to loneliness, exhaustion, and resentment. And, hope does not appear among the positive emotions identified by Hall as characteristic of caring, which included only warmth and love. Finally, Hall emphasizes that care is most often aimed at those with a major physical or mental disability. As we have argued above, other-oriented hope, though often triggered by recognizing another's vulnerability, can involve purely growth-oriented hope directed toward otherwise healthy individuals.

In a more recently developed psychological perspective on caring, Leffel et al. (2008) sought to identify key *moral affective capacities* related to taking care of others. Grouped into four motive foundations of care, the moral affective capacities included guilt, forgiveness, and humility (termed reparation-related capacities); gratitude and pride (termed reciprocity-related); trust, love, and elevation (termed attachment-related); and empathy, compassion/sympathy (termed altruism-related). While no role is given to the capacity of other-oriented hope, such a capacity can be seen as complementing either the attachment- or altruism-related capacities. Vicarious hope (along with trust, love, and elevation) may be another capacity through which our bonds with others can be strengthened, and (along with empathy and compassion/sympathy) may be another capacity through which we help and foster the well-being of others in need.

Wolf (1986) reviews conceptions of caring from a nursing perspective. Based upon a self-report measure of nursing-related care behaviours, the ten highest ranked caring behaviours were: attentive listening, comforting, honesty, patience, responsibility, information provision, touch, sensitivity, respect, and calling the patient by name. Hope is not listed among these top-ranked attributes and, indeed, these attributes focus upon present-oriented care elements rather than a future-orientation toward the care recipient. Mayeroff (1971, as cited in Wolf 1986) does include hope among seven elements of caring, and emphasizes that hope is oftentimes growth-oriented rather than focused only upon alleviation of distress or amelioration of pathology.

Watson (1988) discusses *caring versus curing ethics* within the nursing discipline, emphasizing that the former is a moral ideal and end unto itself, and is a necessary prerequisite to attempts to cure. The caring ethic is described by Watson as being a transpersonal act, thereby constituting a high degree of other-interest, as in the case of other-oriented hope. Finally, in the context of palliative care, Richardson et al. (2012) argue for the simultaneous consideration of caring and empathy that is directed toward patients' hope, thereby encircling several aspects of other-oriented hope including future orientation, focus upon the other, growth-orientation, vulnerability, uncertainty, and limited controllability.

## 6.8 Other-Oriented Hope and Worry

Hope often concerns desires toward alleviating a concern, such as hoping that a child will recover from an illness or hoping that one's car will once again run smoothly. As a result, hope and worry are not entirely separable. Worry has been described as:

> … negatively valenced verbal thought activity. When we worry, we are talking to ourselves a lot about negative things, most often about negative events that we are afraid might happen in the future. (Borkovec et al. 1998, p. 562)

There are several similarities between worry and hope. Although worry can be present- or past-oriented, it often concerns the future, thereby resembling other-oriented hope. Both hope and worry involve a significant degree of uncertainty, emphasize cognitive and emotional processes, and can concern the self or others. With respect to this latter point, the other-regarding and self-regarding features of worry were demonstrated in research in which people who held other-oriented values of benevolence and universalism exhibited worries toward others and society, whereas people who held self-oriented values of power and achievement exhibited worries regarding their own well-being (Boehnke et al. 1998).

Consistent with the idea that the concepts of worry and hope share several features, some have viewed worry and hope as likely to positively co-occur.

Lazarus (1991), for example, says that "hope is yearning for amelioration of a dreaded outcome" (p. 282). Lazarus goes on to argue that even in the absence of a dreaded outcome, the uncertainty associated with hope means that hope typically involves a negative (i.e., worrisome) situation. Lazarus gives the following examples of the confluence of hope and despair:

> ...when we have symptoms of illness, we are anxious but hope that we are not seriously ill; when we face an important exam, we are anxious about a negative outcome but hope that we will not fail; when we see that our stamina is failing in an important race, we are also anxious about not making it to the end but hope that we can. We dispel negative emotional tendencies with hope. (p. 283)

From the point of view of Lazarus (1991), then, the more we worry, the more we are hopeful that the feared events do not occur, ultimately counteracting the worry. Similarly, other-oriented hope would be expected to co-occur alongside other-oriented worry. We may worry that a relative's health is poor, and hope that a recovery is soon to occur. Indeed, Bland and Darlington (2002) identified a positive relationship between other-oriented hope and grieving among family members of a relative with mental illness; that is, the more these family members worried about their loved-one's current circumstances, the more they also experienced hope toward their loved-one's future. And, in the context of mothers of children with severe disabilities, Larson (1998) identified the struggle to balance hope and fear: "In embracing the paradox of their child's disability, mothers attempted to maintain a tenuous hopefulness, somewhere between their fears that the doctors were correct and their hope for a miraculous cure" (p. 871).

Despite similarities between worry and hope and some evidence of their co-occurrence, worry and hope are also distinguishable on several dimensions. Worry is negative in valence whereas hope is positive in valence (although both the uncertainty surrounding hoped-for outcomes and the occurrence of dashed hope involve negative affect; Alarcon et al. 2013; Lazarus 1999; Roseman et al. 1990). Worry involves avoiding undesired outcomes whereas hope is oftentimes directed toward approaching desired outcomes; in this way, worry is more defensive or avoidant whereas hope is more approach-oriented. Moreover, worry is associated with ill-health, whereas hope co-occurs with favourable health status; similarly, worry is associated with depression and hopelessness, whereas hope is a significant correlate of well-being (Snyder 2002).

Congruent with these opposing features of hope and worry, the two may be viewed as inversely correlated. In this case, the more we are hopeful, the less we are likely to worry, and the less we are hopeful, the more we are likely to worry. In line with Fredrickson's (2001) broaden-and-build theory, positive emotions such as hope can mitigate the impact of negative events and the worry they conjure within us, reducing our distress. For example, Mednick et al. (2007) showed that, among mothers of children with Type 1 diabetes, greater (self-oriented) hope was associated with lower (self-oriented) worry. They argue that hope may serve as a protective factor against worry among this population. Ogston et al. (2011) showed a similar relationship among mothers of children with autism or Down syndrome.

Therefore, in this view, hope can be viewed as antagonistic or antithetical to worry; similarly, other-oriented hope and other-oriented worry may oppose each other. Being hopeful toward others may stave off worries about those others; conversely, worrying about others may prevent the occurrence of hope toward those others.

In contrast to the views of hope and worry as either being positively or inversely associated, hope and worry can be seen as independent dimensions underlying behaviour. In this view, people vary in the degree to which they are hopeful, they vary in the degree to which they are prone to worry, and these two aspects of functioning are largely unrelated. (Note that this means that some people may experience both high hope and high worry while others may experience high hope and low worry, as in the above examples). This view is similar to that taken of the relationship between dimensions of functioning characterizing people's level of positive and negative emotion (Watson et al. 1998) and of the relationship between dimensions of functioning characterizing people's level of mental health and their level of mental illness (Keyes 2005). Positive emotion is a dimension of emotional functioning that is independent of negative emotion; people can have a disposition to experience high positive emotion accompanied by any level of trait negative emotion (i.e., high, moderate, low). In a parallel fashion, the psychological dimension of functioning related to the presence of mental health is distinct from that related to the presence of mental illness, such that mental health and mental illness can be viewed as two distinct aspects of people's functioning.

Hope overlaps both with positive emotionality and with positive mental health, whereas worry overlaps both with negative emotionality and with mental illness. Therefore, like these more superordinate dimensions of functioning, the degree to which people are hopeful and the degree to which they are prone to worry may be largely independent aspects of people's functioning: people may be very hopeful and worry a great deal, moderately, or not at all; people may be prone to worry and be very hopeful, moderately hopeful, or hopeless. For example, Ojala (cited in Persson et al. 2011) states, in the context of youth's concerns about environmental destruction, "Young people who are highly worried can also feel positive emotions to high degree, which seems to have a positive impact on both well-being and behaviour (p. 138). This conceptualization of hope and worry as two separable dimensions is also consistent with Barilan's (2012) argument that hope is promotion-focused as opposed to prevention-focused. He says "dealing with suffering and other misfortunes is not at the center of hope" (p. 171); rather, hope aspires toward fulfillment. Aristotle, too, argues that hope focuses more upon the pursuit of good ends rather than avoiding dreaded ones (Gravelee 2000), supporting a conceptual distinction between hope and worry and thereby supporting their relative independence.

**Box 6.2: Hoping-For, Hoping-Against**

Wendy Edey (Larsen et al. 2014) is an experienced registered psychologist who over the past 18 years has explored the use of hope in therapy. Her work commonly includes asking her clients what they hope for. At an appropriate

time, usually early in therapy, she will work with clients to de
list of their hopes. She very often encourages clients to use the
explicitly. Entering therapy, clients are often as aware of what
avoid as what they seek. Clients sometimes enter these early c
with Ms. Edey saying things like, "*I hope to not be so depress[...]*" Seeing these as fearful and avoidant responses, Ms. Edey calls this sort of negative response, 'hoping-against', as in hoping against more depression. Working gently with clients, she encourages them to experiment with the language of 'hoping-for'. Hoping-for responses offer clients the vision of something personally desirable to move toward.

Likewise, *other-oriented* hope and *other-oriented* worry may be two aspects of functioning that are largely independent of each other. Within such a conceptualization, the presence or absence of other-oriented hope is independent of the presence or absence of other-oriented worry. For example, a person holding much hope toward others could also exhibit a great deal of worry toward others, a moderate degree of worry toward others, or be relatively worry-free about others. Similarly, a person who worries a lot about others could also hold high hope toward others, moderate hope toward others, or little hope toward others. Put differently, the absence of other-oriented hope is not synonymous with the presence of other-oriented worry, and the presence of other-oriented worry is not synonymous with the absence of other-oriented hope; rather, the two underlying dimensions of other-oriented hope and other-oriented worry may vary independently of each other. One implication of such a conceptualization is that research on worry and other-oriented worry does not substitute for research on hope and other-oriented hope. Because the two dimensions of functioning (hope and worry) are separable, each needs to be understood in its own right. Thus far, the amount of research devoted to our understanding of worry vastly outweighs that devoted to hope.

In sum, other-interest, altruism, compassion, empathy, love, caring, and worry are all related to, but distinguishable from, other-oriented hope. Other-interest is a broader concept than vicarious hope, subsuming numerous processes concerning our orientation toward others beyond hope per se. Altruism, compassion, empathy, love, caring, and worry are more present-oriented relative to other-oriented hope, are more aimed at alleviation of distress and other negative experiences and less toward the attainment of growth or positive outcomes and, on balance, are more automatically elicited than voluntarily emitted. Overall, we view other-oriented hope as distinguishable from altruism, empathy, compassion, love, caring, and worry but we acknowledge that other-oriented hope is likely to positively correlate with many of these additional psychological concepts. In addition, other-oriented hope, like these other concepts, should also positively correlate with the higher-order concept of other-interest.

## ·erences


Alarcon, G. M., Bowling, N. A., & Khazon, S. (2013). Great expectations: A meta-analytic examination of optimism and hope. *Personality and Individual Differences, 54*, 821–827.

Averill, J. R., Catlin, G., & Chon, K. K. (1990). *Rules of hope*. New York: Springer.

Bailie, T. (2014). *Effects of compassion on vicarious hope and vicarious gratitude*. Unpublished honour's thesis, MacEwan University.

Barilan, Y. M. (2012). From hope in palliative care to hope as a virtue and a life skill. *Philosophy, Psychiatry, and Psychology, 19*, 165–181.

Batson, C. D. (1991). *The altruism question: Toward a social psychological answer*. Hillsdale, NJ: Erlbaum.

Batson, C. D. (2011). *Altruism in humans*. New York: Oxford University Press.

Bergner, R. M., & Ramon, A. (2013). Some implications of beliefs in altruism, free will, and nonreductionism. *Journal of Social Psychology, 153*, 598–618.

Bland, R., & Darlington, Y. (2002). The nature and sources of hope: Perspectives of family caregivers of people with serious mental illness. *Perspectives in Psychiatric Care, 38*, 61–68.

Boehnke, K., Stromberg, C., Regmi, M. P., Richmond, B. O., & Chandra, S. (1998). Reflecting the world "out there": A cross-cultural perspective on worries, values, and well-being. *Journal of Social and Clinical Psychology, 17*, 227–247.

Borkovec, T. D., Ray, W. J., & Stober, J. (1998). Worry: A cognitive phenomenon intimately linked to affective, physiological, and interpersonal behavioral processes. *Cognitive Therapy and Research, 22*, 561–576.

Bovens, L. (1999). The value of hope. *Philosophy and Phenomenological Research, 59*, 667–681.

Brown, S. L., Brown, R. M., & Preston, S. D. (2012). The human caregiving system. In S. L. Brown, R. M. Brown, & L. A. Penner (Eds.), *Moving beyond self-interest: Perspectives from evolutionary biology, neuroscience, and the social sciences* (pp. 75–88). New York: Oxford University Press.

Bruininks, P., & Malle, B. F. (2005). Distinguishing hope from optimism and related affective states. *Motivation and Emotion, 29*, 327–355.

Cassell, E. J. (2002). Compassion. In C. R. Snyder & S. J. Lopez (Eds.), *Handbook of positive psychology* (pp. 434–445). Oxford University Press.

Dambrun, M., & Ricard, M. (2011). Self-centeredness and selflessness: A theory of self-based psychological functioning and its consequences for happiness. *Review of General Psychology, 15*, 138–157.

Davis, M. H. (1983). Measuring individual differences in empathy: Evidence for a multidimensional approach. *Journal of Personality and Social Psychology, 44*, 113–126.

de Waal, F. B. M. (2008). Putting altruism back into altruism: The evolution of empathy. *Annual Review of Psychology, 59*, 279–300.

Eliott, J. A., & Olver, I. N. (2002). The discursive properties of "hope": A qualitative analysis of cancer patients' speech. *Qualitative Health Research, 12*, 173–193.

Fredrickson, B. L. (2001). The role of positive emotions in positive psychology: The broaden-and-build theory of positive emotions. *American Psychologist, 56*, 218–226.

Frimer, J. A., Walker, L. J., Dunlop, W., Lee, B. H., & Riches, A. (2011). The integration of agency and communion in moral personality: Evidence of enlightened self-interest. *Journal of Personality and Social Psychology, 101*, 149–163.

Gerbasi, M. E., & Prentice, D. A. (2013). The Self- and Other-Interest Inventory. *Journal of Personality and Social Psychology, 105*, 495–514.

Goetz, J. L., Keltner, D., & Simon-Thomas, E. (2010). Compassion: An evolutionary analysis and empirical review. *Psychological Bulletin, 136*, 351–374.

Gravlee, G. S. (2000). Aristotle on hope. *Journal of the History of Philosophy, 38*, 461–477.

Hall, J. N. (1990). Towards a psychology of caring. *British Journal of Clinical Psychology, 29*, 129–144.

Hegi, K. E., & Bergner, R. M. (2010). What is love? An empirically-based essentialist account. *Journal of Social and Personal Relationships, 27*, 620–636.

Herth, K. (1993). Hope in older adults in community and institutional settings. *Issues in Mental Health Nursing, 14*, 139–156.

Howell, A. J., Bailie, T., & Buro, K. (in press). Evidence for vicarious hope and vicarious gratitude. *Journal of Happiness Studies.*

Kelly, A. (2007). Hope is forked: Hope, loss, treatments, and AIDS dementia. *Qualitative Health Research, 17*, 866–872.

Keyes, C. L. M. (2005). Mental illness and/or mental health: Investigating axioms of the complete state model of mental health. *Journal of Consulting and Clinical Psychology, 73*, 539–548.

Lapierre, S., Bouffard, L., Dube, M., Labelle, R., & Bastin, E. (2001). Aspirations and well-being in old age. In P. Schmuck & K. M. Sheldon (Eds.), *Life goals and well-being: Towards a positive psychology of human striving* (pp. 102–115). Toronto: Hogrefe and Huber.

Larsen, D. J., Stege, R., Edey, W., & Ewasiw, J. (2014). Working with unrealistic hope or unshared hope in the counselling session. *British Journal of Guidance & Counselling. DOI, 10* (1080/03069885), 895798.

Larson, E. (1998). Reframing the meaning of disability to families: The embrace of paradox. *Social Science and Medicine, 47*, 865–875.

Lazarus, R. S. (1991). *Emotion and adaptation.* New York: Oxford University Press.

Lazarus, R. S. (1999). Hope: An emotion and a vital coping resource against despair. *Social Research, 66*, 653–678.

Leffel, G. M., Fritz, M. E., & Stephens, M. R. (2008). Who cares? Generativity and the moral emotions, Part 3: A social intuitionist "ecology of virtue". *Journal of Psychology and Theology, 36*, 202–221.

Mansbridge, J. J. (1990). On the relation of altruism and self-interest. In J. J. Mansbridge (Ed.), *Beyond self-interest* (pp. 133–146). Chicago: University of Chicago Press.

Mednick, L., Cogen, F., Henderson, C., Rohrbeck, A. A., Kitessa, D., & Streisand, R. (2007). Hope more, worry less: Hope as a potential resilience factor in mothers of very young children with Type 1 diabetes. *Children's Healthcare, 36*, 385–396.

Miller, D. T. (1999). The norm of self-interest. *American Psychologist, 54*, 1053–1060.

Newton, N. J., Herr, J. M., Pollack, J. I., & McAdams, D. P. (2014). Selfless or selfish? Generativity and narcissism as components of legacy. *Journal of Adult Development, 21*, 59–68.

Ogston, P. L., Mackintosh, V. H., & Myers, B. J. (2011). Hope and worry in mothers of children with an autism spectrum disorder or Down syndrome. *Research in Autism Spectrum Disorders, 5*, 1378–1384.

Oman, D. (2011). Compassionate love: Accomplishments and challenges in an emerging scientific/spiritual research field. *Mental Health, Religion, and Culture, 14*, 945–981.

Ortony, A., Clore, G. L., & Collins, A. (1988). *The cognitive structure of emotion.* New York: Cambridge University Press.

Oveis, C., Horberg, E. J., & Keltner, D. (2010). Compassion, pride, and social intuitions of self-other similarity. *Journal of Personality and Social Psychology, 98*, 618–630.

Penner, L. A., & Orom, H. (2010). Enduring goodness: A person-by-situation perspective on prosocial behavior. In M. Mikulincer & P. R. Shaver (Eds.), *Prosocial motives, emotions, and behavior: The better angels of our nature* (pp. 55–72). Washington, DC: American Psychological Association.

Perry, D., Hendler, T., & Shamay-Tsoory, S. G. (2012). Can we share the joy of others? Empathic neural responses to distress vs joy. *Social and Cognitive Neuroscience, 7*, 909–916.

Persson, L., Lundegard, I., & Wickman, P.-O. (2011). Worry becomes hope in education for sustainable development. *Ultbildning & Demokrati, 20*, 123–144.

Rempel, J. K., & Burris, C. T. (2005). Let me count the ways: An integrative theory of love and hate. *Personal Relationships, 12*, 297–313.

Richardson, K., MacLeod, R., & Kent, B. (2012). A Steinian approach to an empathic understanding of hope among patients and clinicians in the culture of palliative care. *Journal of Advanced Nursing, 68*, 686–694.

Roseman, I. J., Spindel, M. S., & Jose, P. E. (1990). Appraisals of emotion-eliciting events: Testing a theory of discrete emotions. *Journal of Personality and Social Psychology, 59*, 899–915.

Sallquist, J., Eisenberg, N., Spinrad, T. L., Eggum, N. D., & Gaertner, B. M. (2009). Assessment of preschoolers' positive empathy: Concurrent and longitudinal relations with positive emotion, social competence, and sympathy. *Journal of Positive Psychology, 4*, 223–233.

Salzburg, S. (1995). *Lovingkindness: The revolutionary art of happiness*. Boston: Shambhala Publications.

Snyder, C. R. (2002). Hope theory: Rainbows in the mind. *Psychological Inquiry, 13*, 1047–1084.

Underwood, L. G. (2009). Compassionate love: A framework for research. In B. Fehr, S. Sprecher, & L. G. Underwood (Eds.), *The science of compassionate love: Theory, research, and applications* (pp. 3–26). Oxford: Wiley-Blackwell.

van Manen, M. (2002). Care-as-worry, or "Don't worry, be happy". *Qualitative Health Research, 12*, 262–278.

Wallace, B. A., & Shapiro, S. L. (2006). Mental balance and well-being: Building bridges between Buddhism and Western psychology. *American Psychologist, 61*, 690–701.

Watson, M. J. (1988). New dimensions of human caring theory. *Nursing Science Quarterly, 104*, 175–181.

Watson, D., Clark, L. A., & Tellegen, A. (1998). Development and validation of brief measures of positive and negative affect: The PANAS scales. *Journal of Personality and Social Psychology, 54*, 1063–1070.

Weingarten, K. (2010). Reasonable hope: Construct, clinical applications, and supports. *Family Process, 49*, 5–25.

Wolf, Z. R. (1986). The caring concept and nurse identified caring behaviors. *Topics in Clinical Nursing, 8*, 84–93.

Zaki, J., & Mitchell, J. P. (2013). Intuitive prosociality. *Current Directions in Psychological Science, 22*, 466–470.

# Chapter 7
# Outstanding Issues, Future Research Directions, Clinical Applications, and Conclusions

## 7.1 General

> *...one important point of optimism that we can take is that perhaps the moral virtue of hope could become much more widespread now than has ever been possible before. So, even if many of us cannot be truly magnanimous with our goods, there are many of us who can now be giving to others with our hopes and our related efforts. And, this is something that should give us all great hope!*
> —Kraemer (2012, p. 14)

Given the nascent nature of research and theorizing on other-oriented hope, there are several outstanding issues that remain to be considered. In this final chapter, we provide a sketch of several such issues: whether there are strengths of character in addition to hope that are directed both to self and others; the nature of the relationship between other-oriented hope and realism; and the status of other-oriented hope as a virtue. We also examine several directions to be taken in future research on vicarious hope, such as the development of a self-report scale of other-oriented hope. Finally, we examine several clinical applications of vicarious hope, arguing that there may be effective routes toward, and value in, its cultivation.

## 7.2 Outstanding Issues

### 7.2.1 *Do Additional Strengths of Character Have Significant Other-Regarding Aspects?*

We argued in Chap. 6 that other-oriented hope can be conceptualized as one manifestation of the broader concept of other-interest. If so, there may be strengths of character beyond hope that also manifest in forms directed toward the interests of others. In this section, we identify several adaptive traits that, despite typically being considered in their self-oriented form, appear to have both self- and



A.J. Howell and D.J. Larsen, *Understanding Other-Oriented Hope*,
SpringerBriefs in Well-Being and Quality of Life Research,
DOI 10.1007/978-3-319-15007-9_7

other-oriented facets. Specifically, in this section we examine the self- and other-oriented manifestations of optimism, gratitude, fairness, leadership, and acceptance. We also consider whether two character strengths normally considered other-oriented, generativity and compassion, can also be viewed as at times manifesting in a more self-oriented manner.

*Optimism,* a concept that overlaps with hope, has been studied with respect to its application to others. Most research on optimism concerns positive expectations held by people regarding their *own* future good fortune or optimistic explanations offered by people regarding reasons for their *own* successful achievements. For example, a large body of research concerns optimistic explanations given by participants for their recent experiences of success and failure on a personal performance task such as an exam (Seligman 1991). In such instances, successes are commonly attributed to stable, global, and internal factors (such as high intelligence) whereas failures are commonly attributed to unstable, specific, and external factors (such as a teacher's ineptitude). In other words, an optimistic outlook pervades the attributions provided for one's own success and failure experiences. This explanatory style has been shown to have significant adaptive consequences for subsequent psychological functioning.

It turns out that many of the optimistic biases that are self-serving also apply to our expectations for others who are close to us. Baumeister and Leary (1995) state that, "Many of the special biases that people exhibit for processing information in ways that favour and flatter themselves are extended to partners in close relationships" (p. 504). For example, research has shown that, among successful couples, the tendency to take credit for success and to attribute failures to outside forces characterizes explanations for spouses' outcomes (Fincham et al. 1987); among distressed couples, this hopeful interpretation of spouses' behaviour is absent. Additionally, in research previously discussed in Chap. 4, Bruininks and Malle (2005) showed that 11 % of optimism-related stories generated by undergraduate students were altruistic in nature. Therefore, while optimism can reflect self-interest, it appears at times also to reflect other-interest.

Recent work has put forth the argument that *gratitude* may, at times, concern appreciation of others' good fortune in addition to one's own good fortune. Emmons and Mishra (2010) define gratitude as "an acknowledgement that we have received something of value from others" (p. 248). Adopting a more encompassing conceptualization of gratitude, Wood et al. (2010) define it as a "life orientation towards noticing and appreciating the positive in life" (p. 891). These conceptualizations of gratitude are congruent with the possibility of a form of gratitude that is other-oriented; that is, if gratitude reflects appreciation for positive events, including others' benevolence, then one might appreciate positive events experienced by others as well as those experienced first-hand.

Howell et al. (in press, a) conceptualize other-oriented gratitude as *the tendency to notice and appreciate the positive in another person's life.* This notion resembles the Buddhist concept of *mudita* (empathic joy) and the concept of *happy-for* emotional reactions described by Ortony et al. (1988), both of which concern the experience of delighting in response to another person's good fortune (see also Chap. 6).

This notion also resembles the concept of *active-constructive responding* (see also Chap. 5), which involves positively responding to another's good fortune in a way that allows the other to capitalize upon a success (e.g., Gable and Reis 2010). Howell et al. found instances of other-oriented gratitude when undergraduate participants were asked to list events for which they were grateful. And, like hope, more other-oriented gratitude was seen when participants were primed to consider themselves or others when they generated their gratitude responses. However, the rate of other-oriented gratitude was significantly lower than the rate of other-oriented hope. Howell et al. speculated that this could reflect several processes: First, potential other-oriented hopes are unlimited in number whereas other-oriented gratitude requires that the desired event has occurred; therefore, there are fewer opportunities for the latter than for the former. Second, there may be more to be gained through other-oriented hope than through other-oriented gratitude; that is, facilitating another's goal attainment through vicarious hope may be more important than appreciating another's already attained goals. Third, it may be less threatening to hope for others' future good outcomes than to celebrate others' current good outcomes; contemplating others' current or past good fortunes invites competing feelings such as envy, which might reduce the ease and frequency with which such forms of gratitude are experienced. For example, we may not appreciate a good friend's success in a performance domain close to our own hearts, in line with Tesser's (1988) self-evaluation maintenance model.

*Fairness* is another character strength that appears to have an other-oriented counterpart. While we can be concerned that we ourselves are treated in a fair and just manner, that concern can also be directed to the extent to which others around us are treated fairly. Research by van den Bos and Lind (2001) showed that people are as sensitive to a lack of procedural fairness experienced by another (*other-oriented justice*) as they are to an injustice experienced directly by the self. Specifically, within the context of a laboratory-based performance task, participants responded with a similar degree of indignity to experimentally manipulated experiences of unfairness experienced by themselves or their research partners. van den Bos and Lind conclude: "There do exist at least some situations in which we can feel the pain of injustice as sharply when others experience it as when we experience it ourselves" (p. 1333).

*Leadership* is yet another character strength that can be directed toward self-interest or other-interest. Williams (2014) argues that positions of leadership and power can enhance the tendency toward the pursuit of self-focused goals, such as the attainment of wealth and prestige. These goals, in turn, reflect traits such as low agreeableness, self-enhancing values, and a view of the self as independent from others. Conversely, those in a position of power who eschew self-focused goals—likely reflecting such personal traits as high agreeableness, self-transcendence values, and a view of oneself as connected with others—will not utilize that power to the betterment of the self but rather will seek to better the welfare of their organization or of their employees or citizens. Therefore, the character strength of leadership can be viewed from either a self-focused or an other-focused perspective, similar to that of self-oriented and other-oriented hope.

We next examine *acceptance* as a positive psychological attribute that likely occurs in both self-oriented and other-oriented variants. According to Williams and Lynn (2010), acceptance involves "an awareness of both the positive and negative aspects of the self and others while maintaining an attitude of positive regard" (p. 6). Therefore, acceptance is conceptualized as applying to internal experiences but also to external experiences, including the experiences of other people. Aspects of acceptance outlined by Williams and Lynn include non-judgment, tolerance, willingness to involve oneself in experience, nonattachment, and non-avoidance. Acceptance toward others may be exhibited through not judging others, being tolerant of others who are perceived as different than oneself, being willing to engage with others, and not avoiding others who might be predicted to displease us or upset us. It would appear, therefore, that acceptance, like hope, can be directed toward the self or toward others. Interestingly, acceptance of the self and acceptance of others are included, respectively, in measures of psychological well-being and social well-being (Keyes 2005), suggesting that both self-acceptance and other-acceptance are considered key aspects of psychological health.

Therefore, there are several strengths of character that, although typically viewed from the standpoint of self-interest, can also be expressed in a manner that emphasizes other-interest. Finally, we consider two character strengths that are normally viewed from the standpoint of other-interest but that have recently been shown also to reflect self-interest. The personal development of *generativity* (see also Chap. 5), deemed originally by Erikson (1974) to be other-regarding, oftentimes involves the co-occurrence of self- and other-regard (McAdams 2013). Frimer et al. (2011) showed that a group of moral exemplars (highly committed and long-standing volunteers) described their personal strivings in a manner that integrated agency (a self-enhancing motive) and communion (an other-enhancing motive; see Chap. 2). Relatedly, Newton et al. (2014) documented a substantial degree of other-regard among middle-aged participants' responses to several questions regarding their futures (including specific questions regarding their hopes). Moreover, by combining such qualitative data with quantitative measures of both generativity and narcissism, the researchers showed that descriptions of the future which included both other-regard *and* self-regard were positively associated with generativity and with narcissism. This pattern of findings suggests that leaving a legacy often reflects both self- and other-interest.

A second example of a positive characteristic that is typically viewed as other-oriented but that has also self-oriented aspects is compassion. Neff (2003) construes the concept of *self*-compassion as:

> …being touched by and open to one's own suffering, not avoiding or disconnecting from it, generating the desire to alleviate one's suffering and to heal oneself with kindness. Self-compassion also involves offering nonjudgmental understanding to one's pain, inadequacies and failures, so that one's experience is seen as part of the larger human experience. (p. 87)

Research has supported the adaptive characteristics of self-compassion. For example, Neff et al. (2007) showed that as self-compassion increases over time, so does well-being. They also showed that self-compassion in response to a personally threatening outcome buffers anxiety. Therefore, just as compassion toward others can be viewed as a psychological strength, so too can self-directed compassion.

Overall, these examples of character strengths which involve other-regard in addition to self-regard buttress the concept of other-oriented hope as a counterpart to self-oriented hope by illustrating that several key psychological attributes are often directed toward the inclusion of others within one's scope of concern. In addition, the final examples, concerning generativity and compassion, remind us that those concepts that have largely been construed from the viewpoint of other-regard may, too, have significant self-regarding aspects. It seems, therefore, that several positive personality characteristics involve directing one's interest both inward toward oneself and outward toward others.

### *7.2.2 Is Other-Oriented Hope Realistic Hope?*

Hope is, at times, disparaged as being nothing more than naïve, *Pollyannaish* thinking engaged in by those wearing rose-coloured glasses. This argument holds that hopeful people are unrealistic in their views toward the future, that they ignore or deny reality, and that they invariably are headed toward disappointment. However, numerous of the definitions and conceptual analyses of hope reviewed in Chap. 3 or Chap. 4 explicitly identify realism as an important dimension of hope (Averillet al. 1990; Benzein and Saveman 1998; Hendricks-Ferguson 1997; Hinds and Gattuso 1991; Morse and Doberneck 1995; Pettit 2004). For example, Dufault and Martocchio (1985) define hope as a "*confident but uncertain expectation of achieving a future good which, to the hoping person, is realistically possible and personally significant*" (p. 380). And, Averill et al.'s (1990) first *rule of hope* is that hope should involve a realistic appraisal of probability. Furthermore, those who have defined or conceptualized other-oriented hope have also explicitly identified the importance of the realistic basis of such hope. Herth (1993) states that "*Hope is an inner power that facilitates the transcendence of the present situation and enables a reality based expectation of a brighter tomorrow for self and/or others*" (p. 146). And, our integrative definition of other-oriented hope which appeared in Chap. 3 states that other-oriented hope is a *future-oriented belief, desire, and mental imagining surrounding a valued outcome of another person that is uncertain but possible*. Therefore, hope theorists and researchers have been quite direct about explicating the role of rational, realistic appraisal as an important, if not necessary, aspect of hope and of other-oriented hope.

Snyder (2002) directly addresses the possibility of so-called *false hope* (see also Snyder et al. 2002), providing reasons to question the portrayal of hope as unrealistic. He argues that people who are high in hope carefully align their hope with the nature of their environment, so that their hope has a strong basis in reality. He notes that high-hope individuals are not less likely to attain their lofty goals compared to low-hope individuals. He portrays those high in hope as responding rationally rather than irrationally to impediments that are experienced along the way, such as by changing goals when it is adaptive to do so rather than persisting indefinitely with the pursuit of goals that are unlikely to be achieved. He further argues that those with extreme distortions of reality tend to be low, rather than high, in hope.

The experimental psychologist Schneider (2001) also argues in favour of a realistic basis for hopeful thinking, pointing out that people have significant leeway in the meaning they extract from experience (termed *fuzzy meaning*) and that they are frequently confronted with experiences involving incomplete information (termed *fuzzy knowledge*). According to Schneider, realistic hope stemming from fuzzy meaning involves attending to and underscoring favourable aspects of one's experience, such as framing an upcoming life event as challenging rather than daunting. Realistic hope stemming from fuzzy knowledge involves hoping for positive experiences in uncertain situations, while being aware of the limits of available information. Schneider further argues that, despite the hope-facilitating leeway afforded by fuzzy meaning and fuzzy knowledge, it is important to engage in 'reality checks', to avoid self-deception, and ultimately to accept what cannot be changed.

Breznitz (1986) also distinguishes between realistic hope and self-deception in the form of denial, arguing that it is most adaptive to combine high hope with low denial. Note that within this perspective, hope and denial are viewed as orthogonal to (or independent of) one another: one can hope in the absence of denial, or one can hope in the presence of denial, with the former seen as more adaptive than the latter. Finally, Davis and Asliturk (2011) review research showing that a realistic orientation toward future outcomes, in which one considers both positive and negative possibilities, is associated with coping more effectively with adversity. They state, "Those with a realistic orientation hope for and direct their efforts toward achieving the best outcome, but they have also mentally elaborated upon other possible outcomes" (p. 104).

Illustrating the issue of the realistic basis of hope within a counselling context, Larsen et al. (2014b) construe unrealistic hope as client hope that is *unshared* by the therapist or others, or is *contested* as to its reasonableness. Based upon case studies of individuals undergoing counselling, Larsen and colleagues argue that client hope may be directed toward outcomes that are unlikely but that are nonetheless highly meaningful. They highlight the therapeutic tactic of working toward *informed hope*, which involves "exploring with the client the supporting and disconfirming evidence for their hope…" (p. 8), and "includes both inviting alternate perspectives while respecting the client's autonomy to choose how to engage with hope" (p. 8). Similarly, within an occupational therapy context, Spencer et al. (1997) discuss a process whereby clients' improbable hope can move toward more realistic hope by identifying and discussing both possibilities for, and limitations on, their future functioning. These client-centered therapeutic approaches are consistent with Schneider's (2001) notion of fuzziness or leeway as to what constitutes reasonable hope, with Breznitz's (1986) notion of hope without denial, and with Davis and Asliturk's (2011) notion of a realistic orientation toward the future.

Another applied domain in which the false versus realistic nature of hope plays out concerns physician honesty in imparting diagnostic and prognostic information to seriously ill patients, on the one hand, and patient hope, on the other. While the provision of accurate information to patients may be seen as undermining their hope, Parker-Oliver (2012) argues for the importance of fully informing patients of the nature of their illness, while at the same time working directly upon their hope. Indeed, according to Parker-Oliver, there is no false hope, because the achievement of what is hoped for is less important than the meaning with which life events are imbued during the process of hoping. There can be no falsity to the extraction of personal meaning from our lived experiences, such that all of us can hope reasonably, even those whose future lived experience is foreshortened.

Similarly, Hall (1990) argues that all living persons should be encouraged to have hope, regardless of how much living remains. She decries that 'the dying' (i.e., those with less fuzzy knowledge than the rest of us concerning a likely timeline for death) are often discouraged from maintaining hope for a cure, for such hope may be viewed as unrealistic. In echoing the views of Fromm (1968) and of Kubler-Ross (1975), Hall speaks forcefully and eloquently of the viewpoint that while we live, we must hope and that "without a future there is no present" (p. 179). Hall identifies the following meanings of hope among those with terminal illnesses, based upon her interviews with HIV-positive individuals and her own experience with metastatic cancer:

1. Having a future life in spite of the diagnosis.
2. Having a renewed zest for life.
3. Finding a reason for living, usually one that was not evident before.
4. Finding a treatment in the professional or alternative care system that one believes will contribute to survival. (p. 183)

From the perspective of Hall (1990), then, hoping right up to the point of death is not false hope; it is the lifeblood of all of us, well or unwell, and for whom death is imminent or (as far as can be predicted) not imminent. As in the framework of Schneider (2001), this example demonstrates that hope reflects ongoing subjectivity or fuzziness regarding the meaning with which one chooses to imbue one's life circumstances and a degree of uncertainty regarding the possibility of a cure as long as one is alive.

In line with this view, Campbell et al. (2010) discuss communication strategies to impart hope to those with terminal illnesses, providing the following example:

> *Patient*: Well, my daughter is getting married in the spring. I need to be there to give her away.
> *Doctor*: That sounds important. I certainly hope you are able to make it to her wedding in the spring, but I'm worried that may not happen.
> *Patient*: It has to.
> *Doctor*: Let's hope for that. And, I'll certainly work with you to meet that goal. What else is important to you? (p. 464)

By supporting patient hope, while at the same time remaining realistic, physicians can help patients to identify what is important to them in the remainder of their lives. In this manner, physicians are operating within the leeway afforded by the necessary presence in such circumstances of both fuzzy meaning and fuzzy information. Importantly, this example also illustrates the issue of realism as it pertains to other-oriented hope, in the form of physician hope toward the patient. By expressing their own hope for patients, physicians strengthen the patient-doctor relationship by directly communicating their concern for their patients' futures and by supporting patient hope. Moreover, as patients are encouraged to hope even under the direst of circumstances, family members of patients will also feel empowered to hope for their loved ones, thereby increasing the support provided to patients and the expression and validation of family members' feelings surrounding their loved ones' circumstances.

Like self-oriented hope, other-oriented hope can be contested and, in extreme instances, such hope may impede coping, such as by encouraging ongoing denial among family members of the objective circumstances faced by their loved one. *Hoping against hope for others* may, at times, be more costly than beneficial. If another's situation is dire, and if that person's future is predictable on the basis of well-documented clinical findings, other-oriented hope regarding, say, a cure for the other's condition is unwarranted (although praying for such outcomes remains a viable option; Parker-Oliver 2002). However, we surmise that such instances are either relatively rare, given the typical uncertainty and ambiguity of the majority of medical circumstances, or relatively temporary, given that short-term disbelief often precedes acceptance of reality. Nonetheless, the contested nature of such hoping may reveal important and meaningful information regarding the experiences of those who temporarily hold such hope as a coping tactic. Indeed, it may be a key indicator of deeply held values and meaning. Finally, hope changes over time and with new information (Larsen et al. 2014b); as a result, unrealistic hope toward others may shift over time, giving way to alternative, seemingly more realistic other-oriented hope. Instead of hoping for a cure, other-oriented hope may come to include hoping for the other's freedom from pain, for the ability to remain at home, or for the ability to enjoy the company of loved ones.

Overall, to the extent that other-oriented hope is characterized by reasonable interpretations and understandings of another's situation, given the uncertainty in arriving at such judgments in complex and ambiguous circumstances, it is likely that such hope will incur more benefits than costs. As an example, a parent of a terminally ill child may, when information about the child's prognosis is unequivocal and when that information is able, over time, to be truly absorbed and understood, abandon previously held hope for their child's survival (i.e., accepting what cannot be changed), and instead adopt new hope targets, such as hoping that the child feels little pain or hoping that the child's remaining time is highly fulfilling. In our view, it is important to attend to, enquire about, and support the vicarious hope of family members as they seek to understand, cope with, and provide support toward their loved ones' challenging circumstances. It is likely that at least some of the lifeblood of hope occurs in the form of other-oriented hope, and that circumstances are never too late or too dire for such hope. Exploring family members' (or therapists' or physicians') hope toward the patient may clarify important decisions, highlight defining family values, and spur on actions toward enhancing the patient's comfort and meeting the patient's needs. It may also facilitate the ability of caregivers both to provide support and to cope with their own distress.

### 7.2.3 Should Other-Oriented Hope Be Viewed as a Virtuous Form of Hope?

A final outstanding issue that we wish to consider is the extent to which other-oriented hope is reasonably viewed as virtuous hope. Arguments favouring the recognition and cultivation of other-oriented hope would be bolstered to the extent that it was understood as a virtuous form of hope.

An attempt to conceptualize hope as a morally redeemable trait was the ambitious work of positive psychology founders Christopher Peterson and Martin Seligman (2004). On the basis of philosophical, theological, and psychological sources, Peterson and Seligman created a taxonomy of 24 strengths of character, conceptualized as comprising six character virtues: wisdom, courage, humanity, transcendence, temperance, and justice. The character strength taxonomy places hope within the virtue of transcendence, the virtue that "allows individuals to forge connections to the larger universe and thereby provide meaning to their lives" (p. 519). Hope, considered alongside related concepts of optimism, future-mindedness, and future orientation, is defined by Peterson and Seligman as "a cognitive, emotional, and motivational stance toward the future" (p. 570). Along with hope, the other character strengths within the transcendence virtue are gratitude, humour, appreciation of beauty and excellence, and spirituality. Research from this perspective has shown that the character strength of hope is associated significantly with life satisfaction (Park et al. 2004; Peterson et al. 2007). Indeed, Snyder (2004) argues that, because the association between hope and life satisfaction is stronger than the association between most other strengths and life satisfaction, hope can be considered to be a particularly important strength of character. Therefore, hope (even in its more common, self-oriented form) is considered a redeemable characteristic of psychological functioning.

Like many other positive psychology concepts, a criticism directed toward hope as it is conceptualized by Peterson and Seligman (2004) is that it is an *empty* concept, held out as a positive attribute independent of the objects or events that are the targets of hope (Fowers 2008). Fowers states, "Hope can be a character strength only if (one's) dreams or plans are truly worthwhile. If my plan is to exploit or enslave others to become fabulously wealthy, my hope can hardly be seen as a character strength (p. 635). And, Billias (2010) argues:

> Surely I can hope for harm to befall my enemy as readily as I can hope for good to come to my beloved, for world peace and for Osama bin Laden to be killed, for a cure for cancer and for chocolate cake for dessert. What does hope have to do with any notion of goodness? (p. 24)

Snyder (2002) explicitly acknowledges the value-neutral aspects of goals pursued in relation to agency and pathways thinking within his theory of hope. He states:

> Hope theory is meant to be neutral in its treatment of the value of the goals selected by people. .. Therefore, because a person has high hope, there is no theoretical premise that prosocial, positive goals are being pursued. (p. 267)

However, Snyder further argues that most hopes will nonetheless be objectively positive in nature, reflecting the reinforcement of positive goal pursuit in society: "… although hope theory is neutral about the value of goals, its actual application takes place in the context of most people having … positively valued goals" (2002, p. 267).

As discussed in Chap. 5, other hope theorists have argued that it is most appropriate to conceptualize hope as aimed at the *betterment* of self or others, or toward socially valued ends (e.g., Averill et al. 1990). While desires or wishes might be aimed at negative or malevolent outcomes, the concept of hope is restricted by some to a focus upon futures which advance the welfare of oneself or others.

Beyond arguments that hope is, typically if not necessarily, oriented to positive futures, the virtuous nature of hope may depend upon the extent to which the target of hope is the self or others. Virtue or morality turns on the degree to which one's behaviour aids or harms others. Along these lines, a number of scholars have asserted that hope is moral to the extent that hope is oriented toward the interests of others and not just to one's own interests. For example, Nunn (2005) defines *virtuous hope* as hope that is directed toward the good of others or the entire community, rather than to the self alone. Interpreting the writings of Augustine of Hippo, Nunn states:

> The prudential good, or, in other words, the rational self-interest, of the person hoping and the good overall, or the good objectively, or the good of the community, do not always coincide … Human beings can hope prudentially in opposition to the 'objective' good, for example, hope in their own selfish interests and to the detriment of the interests of others. (p. 64)

Elsewhere, Nunn (2005) states:

> When hope is practiced as a virtue the prudential hope of the hoper and what they perceive as the objective good will coincide. This is because a virtuous person's desires, judgments, and beliefs are integrated or in harmony with one another and the objective good. (p. 68)

Similarly, Kraemer (2012) argues that ethical hopes are aimed at objectively significant goods, applied universally (i.e., in a disinterested manner to all persons), and linked to dispositions to act accordingly. Kraemer gives as examples of virtuous hopes "hoping for the extermination of malaria, hoping for an end to domestic violence and child-abuse, hoping for world peace, hoping for a better world, even hoping for everyone's salvation" (p. 6). These are, of course, examples of other-oriented hope.

Therefore, there are strong arguments that other-oriented hope plays a significant role in virtue by reason of its distribution of interest among persons beyond the self. Virtuous hope can be viewed as hope that stands to benefit others instead of, or in addition to, the self. In this way, virtuous hope overlaps significantly with vicarious hope.

In contradistinction to vicarious hope, self-oriented hope is often morally neutral, reflecting the fact that self-oriented hope typically neither facilitates nor impedes others' welfare. For example, hoping to perform well on an upcoming exam or hoping to have an enjoyable vacation may have no immediate consequences for the welfare of others around us. Self-oriented hope should therefore not be construed as morally questionable; indeed, even blatantly self-interested ways of thinking or hoping are common and necessary in everyday experience. Nonetheless, this self-orientation requires counterbalancing with attention and concern toward others with whom we live and interact. The philosopher Peter Singer (1981) and social psychologists Brewer and Caporael (1990) acknowledge a tension between self-centered desires and imperatives of social living:

> The shape of human ethical systems is an outcome of the attempt of human societies to cope with this tension between collective reasoning and the biologically based desires of individual human beings. (Singer 1981, p. 147)
>
> Sociality should not be confused with noncontingent altruism. We do not doubt that human beings are vested with a great deal of self-interest, but contend that self-interest is naturally mitigated by identification with groups. (Brewer and Caporael 1990, p. 241)

And, on the basis of their evidence that the dualism between self- and other-interest is surmounted in those who arise to high levels of moral behaviour, Frimer et al. (2011) state:

> … (moral exemplars) defy this dualism by integrating their personal ambitions with their moral convictions, yielding a state of 'enlightened self-interest' in which their own interests become aligned with the interests of others…. (p. 150)

Therefore, other-oriented hope can be viewed as an aspect of ethical or virtuous behaviour, balancing out the natural and necessary propensity to harbour self-oriented hope.

## 7.3 Future Research Directions on Other-Oriented Hope

As reviewed in Chap. 4, evidence for other-oriented hope has accrued in numerous quantitative and (especially) qualitative studies, including those that have examined other-oriented hope among parents, informal caregivers, and formal caregivers. The vast majority of these studies have occurred within a health care context. A smaller number of studies have yielded evidence of other-oriented hope among people in more general contexts. Notably, the majority of evidence for other-oriented hope has arisen indirectly, in that most studies yielding evidence in support of vicarious hope did not set out deliberately to uncover it.

Given the nascent, indirect, and heterogeneous nature of research conducted thus far on other-oriented hope, there are numerous directions for future research on this topic. In this section, we outline several such lines of research. Specifically, we describe the importance of the creation and validation of a self-report measure of other-oriented hope, the necessity for correlational and experimental quantitative research, and the need for further qualitative work on other-oriented hope.

### *7.3.1 Development of a Self-report Measure of Other-Oriented Hope*

Is it possible to measure other-oriented hope with a self-report instrument? There are several reasons to believe that the development of such an instrument will be a fruitful step in forwarding research on other-oriented hope. First, research on *self-oriented* hope has benefitted greatly from the development of various self-report measures of hope, such as Snyder's Hope Scale (Snyder et al. 1996). Many of these scales have yielded evidence for their reliability (e.g., internal consistency, temporal stability) and validity (e.g., their pattern of correlations with measures of convergent and divergent concepts). Such measures have facilitated research on the nomological web of hope, the network of interrelationships between hope and related concepts such as spirituality, gratitude, or well-being. Hope scales have been devised in versions applicable to both adults and children, in versions tapping unidimensional and multidimensional conceptualizations of hope, and in versions that assess hope as a momentary *state* and hope as an individual difference or *trait*. With respect to the latter point, because state-focused versions of hope scales assess the degree of hope experienced at the time of assessment (i.e., acutely), they afford the detection of changes in hope reflecting fluctuating life circumstances or the effects of interventions.

Second, there have been steps toward the creation of self-report measures of other-oriented hope. Wong and Heriot (2007) describe an unpublished, 20-item scale of vicarious hope and vicarious despair, devised within a context of research on childhood illness. Items (e.g., *I generally believe that my child's future will be very active; I often fear that my child will not have the personal support that they need in the future*) concern parents' views toward their child's future. Kopelowicz et al. (2003) devised the Hope for the Patient's Future Scale, consisting of 20 items on which family members rate their level of hope, including *the illness of your family member gets better* and *your family member will be able to develop his/her own goals for the future* (p. 701). Kopelowicz et al. showed that their scale predicts the level of experienced burden among family members of people with schizophrenia. Hinds and Gattuso (1991) describe the development and validation of a measure of hopefulness *for self and others*, the 24-item Hopefulness Scale for Adolescents. These instruments may prove useful as quantitative assessments of parent and family member hope in future research concerning childhood physical and mental illness, and related parental and family challenges.

Third, the opportunity exists to adapt an existing measure of self-oriented hope, converting it to an alternative form tapping other-oriented hope; this approach capitalizes upon the benefits of developing a scale of other-oriented hope upon the platform of an already-established and psychometrically sound scale of self-oriented hope. Reflecting this approach, Redlich et al. (2010) describe an adapted version of Snyder et al.'s (1996) adult State Hope Scale in which items were reworked in order to reflect family members' hope toward their loved one who was experiencing mental illness. And, Coppock et al. (2010) adapted Snyder's scale in order to assess therapists' hope held for their clients. These scales may be useful in future work concerning similar and related contexts.

Fourth, because researchers have successfully developed and validated self-report scales assessing constructs related to other-oriented hope, the development of a scale of other-oriented hope may benefit from approaches taken in the development of these related scales. A good example is the manner in which Gerbasi and Prentice (2013) devised the Self- and Other-Interest Inventory, a reliable and valid measure of the independent dimensions of self-interest and other-interest. In the development of this inventory, items related to self-interest were paralleled in a second scale concerning other-interest. For example, the self-interest item, *I am constantly looking for ways to get ahead*, occurs in parallel form as the other-interest item, *I am constantly looking for ways for my acquaintances to get ahead.* An advantage of this approach to scale development is that the self-oriented scale acts as a comparison or contrast measure in relation to the other-oriented scale. For example, while other-interest was predicted (and shown) to relate positively to empathy, self-interest was predicted (and shown) *not* to relate to empathy (Gerbasi and Prentice 2013). An opposite pattern was found for the prediction of materialism (i.e., materialism correlated with self-interest but not with other-interest), thereby establishing a *differential* pattern of associations among the concepts.

A similar approach could be taken in the development of a measure of other-oriented hope. For example, the self-oriented hope statement *I often hold hope regarding my own future good health* could be paralleled in the other-oriented hope statement *I often hold hope regarding others' future good health.* Devising a number of such statements in both versions would yield symmetrical measures of self- and other-oriented hope. Upon establishing the reliability and validity of such scales, they could be employed both in basic research aimed at furthering our understanding of the two forms of hope and their interrelationship, as well as in applied research in which the two forms of hope could be assessed and compared among particular groups of individuals (e.g., those expected to have low self-oriented hope but higher other-oriented hope), or among those anticipated to experience increases or decreases in one or both kinds of hope.

### 7.3.2 Correlational Research on Other-Oriented Hope

The development and validation of measures of other-oriented hope will spur quantitative research on other-oriented hope, including mapping the web of associations, both convergent and discriminant, among other-oriented hope and related concepts such as compassion, altruism, agreeableness, love, other-interest, environmentally responsible behaviour, and well-being (with which we would predict positive associations) as well as concepts such as narcissism, entitlement, power, self-interest, and materialism (with which we would predict negative associations). As a specific example, it could be predicted that other-oriented hope may show significant relationships with *eudaimonic well-being* (i.e., being fulfilled, or flourishing), whereas self-oriented hope may show significant relationships with *hedonic well-being* (i.e., feeling good; Waterman 1993).

In addition to studies in which individual differences in other-oriented hope are associated with individual differences in other variables, correlational research can also involve comparing *known groups* of individuals who might be expected to differ on their degree of other-oriented hope. For example, long-standing volunteers, long-term informal caregivers, lovingkindness meditation practitioners, and members of the helping professions may be groups expected to harbour a greater degree of other-oriented hope relative to others. A specific target group for research on other-oriented hope is volunteer blood donors. Elster (1990) and Singer (1981) identify blood donation (at least in countries where no payment is made to the donor) as a prime example of altruistically-motivated behaviour. Blood donors may express more other-oriented hope than people who do not donate blood; furthermore, they may identify that their desire to donate blood is motivated by other-oriented hope.

Other-oriented hope could also be assessed among people who differ as a function of age, gender, social class, life stage, or degree of challenge and adversity recently experienced. First, the degree of other-oriented hope could be compared across groups of individuals of various ages (cross-sectional research), and it could be tracked across time within a single cohort (longitudinal research). This would enable the testing of hypotheses concerning, for example, increases in other-oriented hope that might be expected to accompany older age. Second, researchers could examine differences in other-oriented hope among the genders. If women more than men have a *morality of care* (Gilligan 1977), then they may show a heightened degree of other-oriented hope relative to men. This would possibly reflect the greater socialization of other-interest among females relative to males, and would dovetail with gender differences documented for related concepts such as empathy (Eisenberg and Lennon 1983). Third, other-oriented hope could be examined as a function of socioeconomic status. Specifically, there is reason to predict that other-oriented hope will be more prevalent among those with lower socioeconomic status compared to those of higher social standing. Keltner et al. (2014) argue that prosocial behaviour in general may be less costly and more rewarding for members of society who must rely on each other to a greater degree than members who can thrive relatively autonomously. Keltner et al. review evidence consistent with this hypothesis that economic independence reduces prosociality whereas economic interdependence increases it.

Fourth, other-oriented hope could be examined as a function of life stages, to determine whether, for example, it increases during the *generativity versus stagnation* stage of psychosocial development or whether it increases as a function of such experiences as getting married or becoming a parent. Finally, those exposed to adverse experiences, such as a child's illness or a natural disaster, might differ in their other-oriented hope relative to those not having had such experiences. In this vein, there is some evidence of other-oriented hope expressed among those concerned about environmental issues: Ojala (2012) showed that young people involved in environmental organizations in Sweden held hope that social movements would improve the environment for future generations and for other species (see also Persson et al. 2011). Concerning personal experiences of adversity, more research is required on whether other-oriented hope emerges as a function of approaching the end of life. As reviewed in Chap. 4, Herth (1990) showed that other-oriented hope was most frequently observed among elderly individuals who were experiencing significant disability and who required supported living. The expectation of enhanced other-oriented hope during confrontation with profound experiences, such as facing one's own mortality, is compatible with Reed's (2008) theory of self-transcendence, but requires more direct empirical testing. Indeed, Lapierre et al. (1993) provided contrary evidence that a group of very elderly, impaired individuals identified *fewer* aspirations concerning others than did a group of less elderly, unimpaired individuals. This pattern was presumed to reflect the self-related concerns of the older group, such as preservation of their health, suggesting that people's hope may turn toward more basic, self-preservation concerns under adverse personal circumstances.

In the longitudinal form of correlational research (i.e., research following one group over time and comparing their later attributes with their earlier attributes), it would be interesting to examine the long-term sequelae of other-oriented hope. Crocker and Canevello (2012) argue that the adoption of compassionate goals (i.e., goals concerning the welfare of others) can, over time, affect subsequent goals, social functioning, and even personality development. Likewise, it may be that frequently harbouring other-oriented hope predicts later changes in thinking, feeling, and behaviour. Such effects may include improved relationships, lower stress, greater sense of generativity, higher trait agreeableness, higher empathy and compassion, and a higher likelihood of engaging in volunteerism, community activism, environmentally responsible behaviour, and other pursuits associated with improving others' welfare.

Longitudinal research could also fruitfully examine events that follow the *fulfillment* of other-oriented hope. When one's hope for another's welfare is fulfilled, psychological consequences may follow. Showing appreciation for the other person's success is a likely consequence of the fulfillment of other-oriented hope, as in the Buddhist concept of *mudita* (empathic joy) or the related notion of vicarious gratitude (Howell et al. in press, a), described earlier in this chapter.

Boosts in well-being or feelings of relief may also be common experiences when our hope toward others is fulfilled. Similarly, research could examine the consequences of *unfulfilled* other-oriented hope, which may include frustration, distress, and despondency or, where possible, a doubling-up of efforts directed toward ongoing hope for the other or a readjustment of one's hope for the other reflecting more attainable aspirations for them.

In a different vein, the psychophysiological underpinnings of other-oriented hope could be the target of future quantitative research. Keltner et al. (2014) reviewed evidence for the role of several neurophysiological systems underlying prosocial behaviour. Brain structures implicated include circuitry within the prefrontal cortex, orbitofrontal cortex, nucleus accumbens, ventral tegmental area, the periaqueductal gray, the hypothalamus, and the amygdala. These areas are known to play numerous roles in the mediation of emotional responding. Moreover, they are key locations for the neutrotransmission of dopamine (a neurotransmitter heavily implicated in reward responses), serotonin (a neurotransmitter involved in mood modulation, among several other functions), and oxytocin (a neuropeptide recently discovered to be involved in responding with kindness to another's vulnerability or neediness). It is possible that future work may show that variations in the tendency to hold other-oriented hope are associated with variations in the functioning of these nervous system circuits implicated in prosocial behaviour.

### *7.3.3 Experimental Research on Other-Oriented Hope*

On the one hand, experimental research can identify antecedent conditions that exert an *effect* on other-oriented hope; on the other hand, it can identify other-oriented hope as a *cause* of other outcomes. Therefore, experimental research on other-oriented hope can position other-oriented hope as a dependent variable (i.e., a variable that depends on, or is affected by, particular antecedent conditions) or as an independent variable (i.e., a variable, free to be manipulated, that causes particular outcomes).

Research that attempts to experimentally increase or reduce the occurrence of other-oriented hope will elucidate the psychosocial conditions or processes that cause other-oriented hope. For example, recent research examined the impact of momentary increases in compassion on other-oriented hope. Bailie (2014) showed, in yet unpublished work, that the induction of compassion led to a greater frequency of other-oriented hope on a hope-generation task. This finding was interpreted as being in keeping with the other-regarding nature of compassion, and with established effects of compassion such as reduced perceptions of self-other dissimilarity (Oveis et al. 2010). Moreover, additional outcomes related to other-oriented hope have been shown to be enhanced by compassion manipulations: Hutcherson et al. (2008) showed that social connectedness is elevated by a brief (few minute) loving-kindness meditation practice and Wallmark et al. (2013) showed that an 8-week meditation intervention significantly boosted altruism.

One could also experimentally prime either an independent or interdependent self-construal (e.g., Gardner et al. 1999) prior to participants generating a list of hoped-for outcomes in order to determine whether interdependence fosters a greater occurrence of other-oriented hope whereas independence fosters more self-oriented hope. As another example, a state of high or low mindfulness could be induced in order to determine the influence of mindfulness on the occurrence of other-oriented hope, premised on the idea that mindfulness enhances awareness of one's external surroundings, including the needs of others, and on recent findings that mindfulness training enhances prosocial behaviour (Kemeny et al. 2012). These practices suggest useful points of departure for attempting to boost levels of other-oriented hope in clinical settings, as is discussed further below.

As a further example of experimental research in which other-oriented hope serves as a dependent (outcome) variable, and as an example of research wherein two independent predictors of other-oriented hope are simultaneously assessed, research could examine participants' other-oriented hope as a function of the manipulation of both the perceived relationship to another (e.g., by asking people to think about a close friend versus a stranger) and the perceived context (e.g., by depicting the other as in need of support vs. not in need). It might be predicted that close, vulnerable others lead us to experience the greatest degree of other-oriented hope. Such a pattern of findings would improve our understanding of other-oriented hope by showing that relational closeness and perceived vulnerability are two factors that influence it.

In a more applied context, but still concerning factors that might increase other-oriented hope, the manner in which a loved one's illness is cast may have consequences for the degree of other-oriented hope experienced toward that loved one. Hernandez et al. (2013) argue that greater hope among family caregivers occurs when schizophrenia is conceived as falling along a continuum with normal experiences. Similarly, Post (2013) argues that hope for those with dementia is greater if dementia is conceptualized as being *deeply forgetful*. Conceptualizations of disorder that emphasize their continuity with normality may be associated with a greater degree of hope toward those experiencing such disorders, and with lesser other-oriented despair. In experimental research, conceptualizations of a disorder can be varied systematically, permitting the degree of other-oriented hope to be determined as a function of those variations. For example, one could portray schizophrenia as being continuous or discontinuous with normality and examine the effect of this manipulation on the rate of other-oriented hope toward the person depicted, testing the hypothesis that conceptualizing schizophrenia as continuous with normality increases vicarious hope toward those with the disorder.

Experimental manipulations may also be conducted with the aim of *lowering* other-oriented hope. One possibility is that we may not hope for another's success in a performance domain close to our own hearts. In line with Tesser's (1988) self-evaluation maintenance model, people often feel threatened when others perform well in a domain in which they themselves are invested; therefore, hoping for the other's success in such a situation may be unlikely or at least reduced relative to domains unrelated to one's own self-image. Another possibility is that people experiencing lower self-control reserves may exhibit lower other-oriented hope, premised on the finding that self-control depletion causes reduced cooperation with others and increased aggression toward others (DeWall et al. 2005). Other-oriented hope, like the inhibition of aggression, may require cognitive effort aimed at reducing self-interests which compete with simultaneously occurring other-interests.

In addition to experimental studies in which other-oriented hope is measured as a consequence of the variation of antecedent conditions, other-oriented hope can itself be manipulated in order to determine its impact on subsequent functioning. Research aimed at studying the effects of increased other-oriented hope will require ways of manipulating its occurrence. One possibility for the manipulation of levels of other-oriented hope is the use of writing exercises akin to those employed in the domain of gratitude. Gratitude interventions often involve having people write about things for which they are grateful; this exercise is associated with improved well-being (Emmons and Mishra 2010). Similar exercises have recently been applied to hope. Littman-Ovadia and Nir (2014) had participants write down three positive things that they anticipated for the following day, and then to experience and maintain their feelings associated with one of those people or events for a 5-min period. Participants in the control condition engaged in the same exercise, but instructions did not emphasize the *positive* nature of the anticipated events. The exercise was completed once per day over the course of 7 days. Results showed significant changes, from pre- to post-assessment, in the form of reduced negative affect, emotional exhaustion, and pessimism (although not in the form of enhanced positive affect, life satisfaction, and optimism) among participants in the experimental condition relative to those in the control condition. Littman-Ovadia and Nir also qualitatively coded the listed events and activities, categorizing them into four superordinate categories: relationship activities (e.g., activities with family and friends); pleasurable activities (e.g., hobbies, special events); everyday tasks (errands, household chores); and work/school activities (e.g., homework). Participants in the experimental group listed more activities falling into the relationship activities and pleasurable activities categories, whereas those in the control condition listed more activities falling into the everyday tasks and work/school activities categories. In related research, King (2001) showed that writing about one's best possible future caused later boosts in subjective well-being and reductions in physical health complaints, and Quoidbach et al. (2009) showed that leading people to imagine positive events that could happen in the future boosted subsequent happiness relative to asking people to imagine negative or neutral events in the future.

A similar activity could be employed in which people are asked to write about, or imagine, positive events that could happen to *others*. For example, adapting the instructions provided to participants in the Littman-Ovadia and Nir (2014) research described above, participants could be asked to "Think of three good things (items, people or events) waiting for your best friend tomorrow. Write them down. Choose one of them and try to experience and maintain the sincere heart-felt feelings associated with it for 5 min". This activity could be practiced for several days in succession. Such manipulations of other-oriented hope could be examined with respect to their effects on indices of positive psychological functioning. For example, heightened other-oriented hope may cause a boost in well-being, higher degrees of other-interest, improvements in one's mental balance, greater endorsement of compassionate goals relative to self-image goals, and increased experiences of self-transcendence.

Manipulating other-oriented hope may also have effects similar to those associated with *quieting the ego*. Leary et al. (2006) suggest that task performance can be enhanced to the extent that people are able to lower their degree of self-awareness toward a state of functioning called *hypoegoic*. One means of lowering self-awareness may be to activate other-oriented hope. For example, individuals giving a public presentation might be led to focus their hope upon bettering audience members' understanding of the material being discussed as opposed to adulation and accolades directed toward themselves. The inculcation of a mindset of other-oriented hope may yield improved task performance as a result. Similarly, athletes whose hope is directed toward the successful performance of the team as a whole, or toward the pleasure or entertainment of supporters, may perform more optimally than athletes whose hope is focused upon their own performance, their status on their team, or their upcoming contract renewal.

Therefore, there is a place for laboratory-based experimental research on other-oriented hope. However, in order to counter the limitations of such a quantitative research approach, including potentially limited generalizability to real-word conditions, and recognizing the need for responsive, nuanced understandings of this complex construct, there is a necessity also for ongoing qualitative research on other-oriented hope.

### 7.3.4 Qualitative Research on Other-Oriented Hope

The advance of quantitative research on other-oriented hope will ideally be balanced by ongoing work using qualitative, in-depth approaches to understanding other-oriented hope. Given the subjective nature of other-oriented hope, and its occurrence within lived experience, qualitative approaches are vital for its understanding.

As stated above, among the studies yielding evidence of other-oriented hope, the focus of those studies typically was not squarely upon vicarious hope. The field requires qualitative research in which targeted groups of individuals, such as parents and caregivers of those with serious illnesses, are interviewed regarding their *specific* experiences of other-oriented hope. These inquiries would attend to the lived experiences of other-oriented hope and the various contexts within which it is experienced with respect to locations/contexts; relationships; personal histories of holding, offering, and receiving other-oriented hope; developmental experiences and mapping of other-oriented hope; and local and larger social discourses related to other-oriented hope. Researchers can learn from participants' descriptions of other-oriented hope, curious about who research participants (under a variety of contexts) might hope for; the nature and content of those hopes; how that experience of other-oriented hope might have changed over time; how other-oriented hope may have been threatened or fostered; how their own hope may have consequently changed; the value of holding hope for others; and the value of receiving hope from others.

Such work may identify recurring themes among other-oriented hope; the role that vicarious hope plays in the process of coping; strategies employed in real-life circumstances that facilitated the bolstering of other-oriented hope; how other-oriented hope may be employed in therapeutically beneficial ways; and any drawbacks experienced in relation to harbouring hope for others.

Future qualitative research could also examine evidence of other-oriented hope from archived sources. It may be possible to content-analyze written narratives for evidence of other-oriented hope. Because the most commonly recognized understandings of hope are self-oriented, that is, virtually all definitions of hope reflect a self-orientation (Larsen et al. 2014a), it will be important to sensitize qualitative researchers to the possible presence of other-oriented hope in research interviews and texts. Our research for this book suggests that other-oriented hope, though a seemingly new phenomenon, may have been laying-in-wait for researchers to 'discover' the threads of its existence across numerous published research texts. The same is likely to be so of various qualitative data sources when a researcher is attuned to its possible presence.

Sources of such narrative material could include daily journals and correspondence in the form of letters or emails. Published narratives, such as biographies and speeches, could also be parsed for evidence of other-oriented hope. Such an approach would afford the advantage of uncovering spontaneous occurrences of vicarious hope under naturalistic conditions. As an example of the analysis of hope-related content from archived material, Larsen and colleagues (e.g., Larsen et al. 2008) describe the use of Interpersonal Process Recall in their studies of hope within the counselling context, in which audio- and video-recorded therapy sessions are reviewed on later occasions with the counsellor or the client in order to identify and understand key counselling processes. During playback of the target session, the client or counsellor is interviewed about what was taking place at each therapeutic moment and how it was experienced. This approach could be applied to the identification and interpretation of other-oriented hope within counselling settings. It could also be employed in related circumstances, such as physician-patient or nurse-family interactions surrounding discussions of critical illness, or parent-teacher interactions surrounding discussions of children who are struggling in the classroom setting.

Mixed-methods research, combining quantitative and qualitative approaches, may be especially fruitful in furthering the understanding of other-oriented hope. Howell et al. (in press, a) showed that, among young adults, a quantitative measure of empathic concern correlated with the frequency of other-oriented hope appearing in written statements on a hope-generation task. Other recent research has used even richer qualitative descriptions of hope, linking information derived from those descriptions with quantitatively measured attributes (e.g., Newton et al. 2014). Researchers such as Lapierre et al. (2003) and Newton et al. (2014) have established elaborate procedures for reliably and validly coding other-oriented hope within lengthy narratives describing future aspirations. We foresee the further development of such approaches as a key means of forwarding an understanding of other-oriented hope that is deeply informed by first-hand experiences.

It would also be valuable to conduct mixed-method studies in which respondents identify the characteristics of their experiences of other-oriented hope, and these descriptions are compared with descriptions of their experiences of related phenomena, including instances of empathy, compassion, or caring. In Chap. 3, we described fruitful research by Bruininks and Malle (2005) and by Roseman et al. (1990) in which respondents' experiences of hope were contrasted with their experiences of such related phenomena as optimism, joy, and wishing. Moreover, Averill et al. (1990) used a similar approach which permitted comparisons of attributes of *altruistic hope* with hope that was not aimed at others' welfare. Applied to the investigation of other-oriented hope, these approaches could yield informative insights into the unique and overlapping aspects of the lived experience of vicarious hope and other forms of other-interest.

Qualitative research could also follow-up upon intriguing findings concerning other-oriented hope that require further elucidation. As one example, Schutta and Burnett (2000) found that only one of eight terminally ill cancer patients who participated in a phase I clinical trial (i.e., trials aimed at testing drug toxicity) identified the hope of benefitting future patients through their participation, despite what is presumably a high likelihood of such a benefit accruing; conversely, all participants identified the hope of personal therapeutic benefit, despite the low likelihood of such benefit. This intriguing pattern of findings, pointing to a low occurrence of other-oriented hope among people engaging in seemingly prosocial behaviour, suggests that follow-up work on this topic is needed. For example, it is not clear how hope was probed or elicited, whether a greater endorsement of benefit to others would have occurred if participants were asked directly about such benefits, or how this context might differ from that involving, say, the donation of blood.

## 7.4 Clinical Applications

To the extent that other-oriented hope is seen as having positive consequences for the bearer and target of that hope, and for their relationship (as described in Chap. 5), or to the extent that other-oriented hope is seen as being a virtuous form of hope regardless of its instrumental consequences, the cultivation of other-oriented hope can be considered a meaningful therapeutic goal. How can other-oriented hope be boosted among counselling or therapy clients?

Frank (1968) was one of the first to argue for the importance of the role of hope in client therapeutic response, and the role of the therapist in instilling such hope. Based upon his review of the early research pertinent to this topic, Frank concludes that "…aspects of the therapeutic situation which arouse or strengthen the patient's hopes of relief are positively correlated with short-term improvement in a significant proportion of patients" (pp. 393–394). Orne (1968) concurred with Frank's assessment of the importance of hope in psychotherapy, arguing that hope reflects belief in the possibility of change, belief in the efficacy of treatment, and belief in the ability of the therapist. More recently, Snyder et al. (2000) also described the role of hope in psychotherapy, emphasizing the importance of goal-setting, agency beliefs, and pathways thinking for clients who may experience despondency with respect to their ability to meet their own goals. To summarize the literature concerning the psychotherapeutic focus upon hope, Weis and Speridakos (2011) conducted a meta-analysis on 27 studies that employed strategies to enhance hope among both mental health clients and community members. They reported modest effects of such psychotherapy on measures of hope and life satisfaction, but not on measures of psychological distress. The authors caution that effects were relatively small in comparison to other psychoeducational or psychotherapeutic interventions. Since most studies of hope-focused interventions have adopted the goal-setting framework of Snyder (2002), it is possible that larger effects may accrue with interventions adopting a broader view of hope (e.g., Larsen et al. 2007) within the psychotherapeutic context.

Indeed, other approaches to the incorporation of hope into counselling have embraced a more multidimensional view of hope and, as a result, a lessened focus upon goal setting, agency beliefs, and pathways thinking. For example, Spencer et al. (1997) describe an approach to working with client hope that considers the cognitive, affective, and spiritual aspects of hope, and which integrates goal setting and goal adaptation with a more holistic focus upon understanding hope within the context of the client's life story. Dufrane and Leclair (1984) adopt an existential therapeutic framework for understanding the role of hope in the counselling process, arguing that "the development of hope is contingent upon the attribution of meaning that allows for change and at least some flexibility in the view of the problem situation" (p. 37). Benzein and Saveman (2008) describe a brief intervention applied to couples in which one person had advanced cancer. Nurses engaged the couples in hope-focused conversations across three sessions. Interviews with six couples revealed that the intervention fostered their ability to cope and unburden themselves within a trusting relationship.

As another example, Howell et al. (in press, b) describe a therapeutic approach which adopts Dufault and Martocchio's (1985) model of hope as a framework for structuring hope-focused interventions and for interpreting hope in session. The therapeutic structure employs a variety of techniques drawing primarily on narrative therapeutic (Edey and Jevne 2003; Edey et al. 1998; Larsen et al. 2014b) and psychoeducational approaches. Applied to clients with chronic pain, the group intervention focused on eliciting and magnifying various counter-stories from participants, stories within which chronic pain did not dominate and wherein hope was evident, visible, and tangible in each participant's own experience. As hopeful experiences and stories were revealed during group sessions, facilitators sought to equip participants with the means to generalize learning and awareness to settings beyond the group experience. Results of two studies evaluating this intervention demonstrated significant changes from pre- to post-treatment on such measures as well-being, hope, pain acceptance, and pain catastrophizing.

These integrative, multidimensional approaches to the incorporation of hope-focused therapeutic approaches could be adapted to incorporate a focus upon other-oriented hope. Examples of other-oriented hope could be elicited from clients as a means of illustrating the presence of hope in an otherwise challenging circumstance. The solicitation of personal stories that counter hopelessness could purposely include counter-stories wherein hope was present in an other-oriented form and wherein personal functioning was heightened (e.g., feelings of well-being) in relation to such hope. By paying greater attention to hope directed toward others that persisted despite trying personal circumstances, clients may come to view vicarious hope as a means of capitalizing upon the benefits of hope when self-oriented hope is compromised.

Additional therapeutic distinctions can be borne in mind when it comes to incorporating a focus on hope and other-oriented hope within the counselling process. For example, the qualitative research of Larsen and colleagues (Larsen et al. 2007; Larsen and Stege 2010a, b) showed that therapists can adopt either an implicit or an explicit focus upon hope. In the case of implicit hope, the focus upon hope is indirect, as in the example of a therapist working together with a client to elucidate what an optimal future would look like to the client without referring directly to client hope. In the case of explicit hope, the focus upon hope is direct, as in the example of a therapist working together with a client to identify experiences of high hope, experiences of low hope, and patterns of thinking, feeling, and behaving that appear to be related to such experiences. Larsen and colleagues view *hope work* as part of a general psychotherapeutic framework in which hope plays a central role, either through its direct application or through less direct exploration, in facilitating client progress and growth.

The distinction between implicit and explicit hope work in counselling could apply equally to therapeutic work on other-oriented hope. A therapist could skillfully explore such hope either in an indirect or a direct manner, thereby revealing potentially important therapeutic themes such as the quality of the client's relationships with others, the ease or difficulty with which they identify hope-for-another, and the presence of impediments to other-oriented hope. The client's experience of being the target of others' hope could also be explored; moreover, hope shared between therapist and client could form part of the therapeutic focus upon other-oriented hope.

Additional counselling techniques may also foster hope toward others. Hollis et al. (2007) discuss the role of hope in healing among clients low in hope. They argue that *action* on behalf of the client can be fruitfully aimed at aiding others:

> Action can often focus on a client's need to make things easier or better for family and friends or to serve others … Such activities provide opportunities to satisfy 'me' goals, that of helping others, by thinking of 'we' goals, what others need, and to widen the scope of hope to include hope for loved ones. (p. 54)

One of the advantages of Hollis et al.'s (2007) focus upon actions-for-others is that such work capitalizes upon the known benefits of *behavioural activation* interventions in clinical and counselling contexts. These interventions involve mobilizing the client to re-engage in activities that in the past brought them pleasure and accomplishment. According to a meta-analysis, behavioural activation interventions lead to substantive gains in the area of life satisfaction or well-being (Mazzucchelli et al. 2010). To our knowledge, behavioural activation that directly encourages activity in the service of others has yet to be studied. Such an intervention may be particularly impactful, given that it would combine behavioural engagement (e.g., increased access to positive reinforcement), increased social connectedness, reduced focus upon the self, and enhanced consideration of others. Moreover, such an intervention would capitalize upon evidence that volunteering to help others can significantly benefit the volunteer's well-being (e.g., Son and Wilson 2012; Thoits and Hewitt 2001).

In addition to these means of working with other-oriented hope in a counselling context, *group work* adds additional ways in which client hope toward others may be explored. A unique feature of the group counselling context is that clients may begin to hold hope concerning the well-being of fellow group members. So, just as group cohesion, modeling, and universality may benefit client progress within group therapy contexts (Yalom 1998), the process of coming to hope for fellow group members may be yet another route toward client improvement. Recipients of such hopeful support from fellow group members stand to benefit from an increased sense of social support and belongingness. The possible relationships between group cohesion, belonging, well-being, and other-oriented hope have yet to be explored. Those conveying such other-oriented hope may benefit from a reduced focus upon the self; such self-focused attention often characterizes mental health clients and may play a role in maintaining maladaptive functioning (Ingram 1990). Alternatively, learning various ways of orienting to others, including the fostering of other-oriented hope, may serve to support adaptive functioning.

**Box 7.1: Group Therapy and Other-Oriented Hope**

Important clinical research extends beyond the identification of other-oriented hope in individual therapy. Irving Yalom (e.g., Yalom 1998; Yalom and Laszcz 2005) was amongst the first to identify hope and other key factors such as cohesion as therapeutic mechanisms within group treatment. Recent research highlights the potentially important role that other-oriented hope plays in group treatment.

While researching group therapy for those with chronic pain (Larsen et al. 2014a), I (D. L.) became acutely aware of how group members intentionally (though often silently) held hope for others in the group. The focus of this group for people with chronic pain was on hope and strengths. The goal of the group was to draw attention to these experiences and help group members apply them in meaningful ways to their own lives. After the third group session of six in the structured group sequence, we interviewed clients to learn about what they were experiencing in the treatment. Clients told us that as they listened to others they often invested in hoping for their peers. Indeed, clients made numerous unsolicited references to other-oriented hope, comments like, "*I was hopeful for him that he continues his commitment to what he's doing*". Other-oriented hopes were often specific to the difficulty a peer was experiencing. One group member, Cynthia reflected, "*that's too bad because she made us all laugh. She was laughing and now she's back to being sad. Well, hopefully she'll get back up there. Cause it [laughter] is there. She can do it.*" Other-oriented hopes were often quite specific and practical, as well. Responding to a group member who spoke about how playing guitar gave her hope, Becca, volunteered, "*I hope she goes and plays her guitar ... my hope is that she plays her guitar.*" Further, Dahlia offered a short description of chair yoga, explaining during her research interview, "*I really wanted to hopefully give her something to try.*"

Bearing witness to others' hopes, particularly in a caring atmosphere like a classroom, school, friendship, or even group therapy, may naturally incline us toward other-oriented hope. On the other hand, close relationships themselves may offer safe spaces to share personal hopes while others join us by hoping for us as well.

With respect to additional practices that may facilitate other-oriented hope, research reviewed above suggests that the clinical use of meditation may be one route through which greater degrees of vicarious hope can be attained. For example, meditation aimed at cultivating *mudita* (empathic joy), in which one contemplates another's joy, includes a variation in which the focus of contemplation is another's *anticipated* or *future* joy, in line with the idea of other-oriented hope (Buddhaghosa 1995). The use of meditation to bolster other-oriented hope may have beneficial effects on clinical outcomes such as increased well-being, reduced negative emotionality, decreased self-focused attention, and improved sense of belongingness with others. Similarly, the writing or imagination exercises described above as routes through which other-oriented hope can be induced could be transferable to the clinical setting. Having clients write down their other-oriented hope, both in-session and between-sessions, may be a means of improving client functioning. Or, analogous to the idea of a *gratitude visit*, wherein one directly expresses one's gratitude to another, it would not be unreasonable to conceive of a *hope visit* in which one conveys one's hope toward another. Not only may this generate positive feelings in the recipient of such expression of other-oriented hope, but such acts may have the consequence of positive psychological outcomes for the bearer of such hope and for the relationship between the two parties. Clearly, research validating the benefits of such practices is required before being applied in the clinical context.

## 7.5 Conclusions

> *We hope that our friend's test results will be good, we hope that no one was injured in yesterday's fire, and so on.*
> —McGeer (2004, p. 103)

In this monograph, we have sought to scrutinize the emerging concept of other-oriented or vicarious hope, a concept reflected in everyday, frequently occurring examples such as those by McGeer quoted above, and in profound examples such as the one recounted by Frankl at the outset of this book. In Chap. 1, we introduced the concept and scope of other-oriented hope in general terms, setting the stage for the remainder of the book. In Chap. 2, we forwarded the case for other-oriented hope as a form of prosocial behaviour, or behaviour revealing our interest in others. In Chap. 3, we extensively reviewed the concept and attributes of hope in order to flesh-out the concept of other-oriented hope, with the latter defined as *future-oriented belief, desire, and mental imagining surrounding a valued outcome of another person that is uncertain but possible.* Chap. 4 constituted a review of research, both qualitative and quantitative in nature, that revealed evidence for other-oriented hope, whether by design or more coincidentally. We considered causes and consequences of other-oriented hope in Chap. 5, wherein we also situated other-oriented hope within existing theoretical frameworks emphasizing other-interest, self-transcendence, mental balance, and compassionate goals. In Chap. 6, we underscored similarities and differences between other-oriented hope and related concepts of other-interest, altruism, compassion, empathy, love, caring, and worry. Finally, in the current chapter we identified several outstanding issues, future research directions, and clinical applications concerning other-oriented hope.

**Box 7.2: Last Reflection on Hope**

As you have read this book, you may have become increasingly sensitized to use of the word 'hope' in everyday life. You might notice its very common use in print and even in advertising. Researchers call this *folk language*, our everyday use of the word. As a research participant once told me, once you starting thinking about hope, you notice it everywhere. It's like buying a red car and noticing that they are far more prevalent than you once thought.

Over the years, I (D. L.) have become more accustomed to this complex interplay between the academic study of hope and its everyday and explicit appearance in life. Regularly I receive email messages from family, students, and colleagues. *Hope you had a good vacation. Hope you have fun this weekend. Hope you're feeling better soon.* Before I began researching hope, I offered these kindly salutations to others at least a liberally as others offered them to me. However, when I began researching hope, I became increasingly sensitized to the complexity of the word. I became quite confounded for a time, trying to determine the appropriate use of the word and I stopped sharing salutations like, "*Hope you enjoy your holiday*!" altogether. I wanted to be sure that I was genuine in my offering. Somehow my academic self hadn't quite reconciled with my everyday 'folk' self.

Over the years, I have come to understand these little phrases as more important than I once did. Discourse researchers (e.g., Wetherell et al. 2001) encourage a close look at our use of language and the meanings and social contexts it both reflects and shapes. I have come to understand these seemingly simple salutations as meaningful expressions of a kindly other-orientation, an orientation of which I am often the fortunate recipient. Just yesterday, I received a note from a colleague, "*Hope all's well*!" Though my well-wisher had no particular ability to create any specific outcome for me, she took a moment to invest a thought for my welfare and the time to share that thought with me. As I reflect on this, her simple action alone offers me both a better present and hope for a good future, a future enriched with people who care for my well-being. Perhaps we are all fortunate to have this simple means of offering the same to others.

With these final thoughts, we close the book with our sincerest hope that readers will have been moved to consider the overlooked concept of other-oriented hope. We could not be more pleased than if this monograph spurs on more qualitative and quantitative research on other-oriented hope across numerous academic disciplines, including research on the application of other-oriented hope to the clinical context, and that it heightens awareness of the potential role of other-oriented hope, both as givers and receivers of it, in the lives well-lived of our clients, students, and loved ones.

## References

Averill, J. R., Catlin, G., & Chon, K. K. (1990). *Rules of hope*. New York: Springer.

Bailie, T. (2014). *Effects of compassion on vicarious hope and vicarious gratitude*. Unpublished honour's thesis, MacEwan University.

Baumeister, R. F., & Leary, M. R. (1995). The need to belong: Desire for interpersonal attachments as a fundamental human motivation. *Psychological Bulletin, 117*, 497–529.

Benzein, E., & Saveman, B. I. (1998). Nurses' perception of hope in patients with cancer: A palliative care perspective. *Cancer Nursing, 21*, 10–16.

Benzein, E., & Saveman, B. I. (2008). Health-promoting conversations about hope and suffering with couples in palliative care. *International Journal of Palliative Nursing, 14*, 439–445.

Billias, N. (2010). Hope as a moral virtue. *At the Interface/Probing the Boundaries, 68*, 17–27.

Brewer, M. B., & Caporael, L. R. (1990). Selfish genes vs. selfish people: Sociobiology as origin myth. *Motivation and Emotion, 14*, 237–243.

Breznitz, S. (1986). The effect of hope on coping with stress. In M. H. Appley & R. Trumbull (Eds.), *Dynamics of stress: Physiological, psychological, and social perspectives* (pp. 295–306). London: Plenum Press.

Bruininks, P., & Malle, B. F. (2005). Distinguishing hope from optimism and related affective states. *Motivation and Emotion, 29*, 327–355.

Buddhaghosa, B. (1995). *The path of purification*. Seattle, WA: Buddhist Publication Society.

Campbell, T. C., Carey, E. C., Jackson, V. A., Saraiya, B., Yang, H. B., Back, A. L., & Arnold, R. M. (2010). Discussing prognosis: Balancing hope and realism. *The Cancer Journal, 16*, 461–466.

Coppock, T. E., Owen, J. J., Zagarskas, E., & Schmidt, M. (2010). The relationship between therapist and client hope with therapy outcomes. *Psychotherapy Research, 20*, 619–626.

Crocker, J., & Canevello, A. (2012). Consequences of self-image and compassionate goals. *Advances in Experimental Social Psychology, 45*, 229–278.

Davis, C. G., & Asliturk, E. (2011). Toward a positive psychology of coping with anticipated events. *Canadian Psychology, 52*, 101–110.

DeWall, C. D., Baumeister, R. F., Stillman, T. F., & Gailliot, M. T. (2005). Violence restrained: Effects of self-regulation and its depletion on aggression. *Journal of Experimental Social Psychology, 43*, 62–76.

Dufault, K., & Martocchio, B. C. (1985). Hope: Its spheres and dimensions. *Nursing Clinics of North America, 20*, 379–391.

Dufrane, K., & Leclair, S. W. (1984). Using hope in the counseling process. *Counseling and Values, 29*, 32–41.

Edey, W., & Jevne, R. F. (2003). Hope, illness, and counselling practice: Making hope visible. *Canadian Journal of Counselling, 37*, 44–51.

Edey, W., Jevne, R., & Westra, K. (1998). *Key elements of hope-focused counselling: The art of making hope visible*. Edmonton, AB: Hope Foundation of Alberta.

Eisenberg, N., & Lennon, R. (1983). Sex differences in empathy and related capacities. *Psychological Bulletin, 94*, 100–131.

Elster, J. (1990). Selfishness and altruism. In J. J. Mansbridge (Ed.), *Beyond self-interest* (pp. 44–53). Chicago: University of Chicago Press.

Emmons, R. A., & Mishra, A. (2010). Why gratitude enhances well-being: What we know, what we need to know. In K. M. Sheldon, T. B. Kashdan, & M. F. Steger (Eds.), *Designing positive psychology* (pp. 248–262). Oxford: University Press.

Erikson, E. H. (1974). *Dimensions of a new identity*. New York: Norton.

Fincham, F. D., Beach, S. R., & Baucom, D. H. (1987). Attribution processes in distressed and nondistressed couples: 4. Self-partner attribution differences. *Journal of Personality and Social Psychology, 52*, 739–748.

Fowers, B. J. (2008). From continence to virtue: Recovering goodness, character unity, and character types for positive psychology. *Theory & Psychology, 18*, 629–653.

Frank, J. (1968). The role of hope in psychotherapy. *International Journal of Psychiatry, 5*, 383–395.

Frimer, J. A., Walker, L. J., Dunlop, W., Lee, B. H., & Riches, A. (2011). The integration of agency and communion in moral personality: Evidence of enlightened self-interest. *Journal of Personality and Social Psychology, 101*, 149–163.

Fromm, E. (1968). *The revolution of hope*. New York: Harper & Row.

Gable, S. L., & Reis, H. T. (2010). Good news! Capitalizing on positive events in an interpersonal context. *Advances in Experimental Social Psychology, 42*, 195–257.

Gardner, W. L., Gabriel, S., & Lee, A. Y. (1999). "I" value freedom, but "we" value relationships: Self-construal priming mirrors cultural differences in judgment. *Psychological Science, 10*, 321–326.

Gerbasi, M. E., & Prentice, D. A. (2013). The self- and other-interest inventory. *Journal of Personality and Social Psychology, 105*, 495–514.

Gilligan, C. (1977). In a different voice: Women's conceptions of care and morality. *Harvard Educational Review, 47*, 481–517.

Hall, B. A. (1990). The struggle of the diagnosed terminally ill person to maintain hope. *Nursing Science Quarterly, 3*, 177–184.
Hendricks-Ferguson, V. (1997). An analysis of the concept of hope in the adolescent cancer patient. *Journal of Pediatric Oncology Nursing, 14*, 73–80.
Hernandez, M., Barrio, C., & Yamada, A.-M. (2013). Hope and burden among Latino families of adults with schizophrenia. *Family Process, 52*, 697–708.
Herth, K. (1990). Fostering hope in terminally-ill people. *Journal of Advanced Nursing, 13*, 1250–1259.
Herth, K. (1993). Hope in older adults in community and institutional settings. *Issues in Mental Health Nursing, 14*, 139–156.
Hinds, P. S., & Gattuso, J. (1991). Measuring hopefulness in adolescents. *Journal of Pediatric Oncology Nursing, 8*, 92–94.
Hollis, V., Massey, K., & Jevne, R. (2007). An introduction to the intentional use of hope. *Journal of Allied Health, 36*, 52–56.
Howell, A. J., Bailie, T., & Buro, K. (in press, a). Evidence for vicarious hope and vicarious gratitude. *Journal of Happiness Studies.*
Howell, A. J., Jacobson, R., & Larsen, D. J. (in press, b). Enhanced psychological health among chronic pain clients engaged in hope-focused group counselling. *The Counseling Psychologist.*
Hutcherson, C. A., Seppala, E. M., & Gross, J. J. (2008). Loving-kindness meditation increases social connectedness. *Emotion, 8*, 720–724.
Ingram, R. E. (1990). Self-focused attention in clinical disorders: Review and a conceptual model. *Psychological Bulletin, 107*, 156–176.
Keltner, D., Kogan, A., Piff, P. K., & Saturn, S. R. (2014). The sociocultural appraisals, values, and emotions (SAVE) framework of prosociality: Core processes from gene to meme. *Annual Review of Psychology, 65*, 423–460.
Kemeny, M. E., Foltz, C., Cavanagh, J. F., Cullen, M., Giese-Davis, J., Jennings, P., et al. (2012). Contemplative/emotion training reduces negative emotional behavior and promotes prosocial responses. *Emotion, 12*, 338–350.
Keyes, C. L. M. (2005). Mental illness and/or mental health: Investigating axioms of the complete state model of mental health. *Journal of Consulting and Clinical Psychology, 73*, 539–548.
King, L. A. (2001). The health benefits of writing about life goals. *Personality and Social Psychology Bulletin, 27*, 798–807.
Kopelowicz, A., Zarate, R., Gonzalez Smith, V., Mintz, J., & Liberman, R. P. (2003). Disease management in Latinos with schizophrenia: A family-assisted, skills training approach. *Schizophrenia Bulletin, 29*, 211–227.
Kraemer, E. (2012). On hope as a moral virtue. In *Presented at Hope: A Conference on the Theological Virtues*. La Crosse, Wisconsin, USA.
Kubler-Ross, E. (1975). *Death: The final stage of growth*. Englewood Cliffs, NJ: Prentice-Hall.
Lapierre, S., Bouffard, L., & Bastin, E. (1993). Motivational goal objects in later life. *International Journal of Aging and Human Development, 45*, 287–303.
Larsen, D., Edey, W., & Lemay, L. (2007). Understanding the role of hope in counseling: Exploring the intentional uses of hope. *Counseling Psychology Quarterly, 20*, 401–416.
Larsen, D., Flesaker, K., & Stege, R. (2008). Qualitative interviewing using interpersonal process recall: Investigating internal experiences during professional-client conversations. *International Journal of Qualitative Research, 7*, 18–37.
Larsen, D. J., & Stege, R. (2010a). Hope-focused practices during early psychotherapy sessions: Part I: Implicit approaches. *Journal of Psychotherapy Integration, 20*, 271–292.
Larsen, D. J., & Stege, R. (2010b). Hope-focused practices during early psychotherapy sessions: Part II: Explicit approaches. *Journal of Psychotherapy Integration, 20*, 293–311.
Larsen, D., King, R., Stege, R., & Egeli, N. (2014a). *Clients' experiences of hope in a hope strengths-based group activity for individuals with chronic pain*. Unpublished manuscript.
Larsen, D. J., Stege, R., Edey, W., & Ewasiw, J. (2014b). Working with unrealistic hope or unshared hope in the counselling session. *British Journal of Guidance & Counselling*. doi:10.1080/03069885.2014.895798.

Leary, M. R., Adams, C. E., & Tate, E. B. (2006). Hypo-egoic self-regulation: Exercising self-control by diminishing the influence of the self. *Journal of Personality, 74*, 1803–1831.
Littman-Ovadia, H., & Nir, D. (2014). Looking forward to tomorrow: The buffering effect of a daily optimism intervention. *Journal of Positive Psychology, 9*, 122–136.
Mazzucchelli, T. G., Kane, R. T., & Rees, C. S. (2010). Behavioral activation interventions for well- being: A meta-analysis. *Journal of Positive Psychology, 5*, 105–121.
McAdams, D. P. (2013). The positive psychology of adult generativity: Caring for the next generation and constructing a redemptive life. In J. D. Sinnott (Ed.), *Positive Psychology: Advances in Understanding Adult Motivation* (pp. 191–205). New York: Springer.
McGeer, V. (2004). The art of good hope. *Annals of the American Academy of Political and Social Science, 592*, 100–127.
Morse, J. M., & Doberneck, B. (1995). Delineating the concept of hope. *Journal of Nursing Scholarship, 27*, 277–285.
Neff, K. D. (2003). Self-compassion: An alternative conceptualization of a healthy attitude toward oneself. *Self and Identity, 2*, 85–102.
Neff, K. D., Kirkpatrick, K. L., & Rude, S. S. (2007). Self-compassion and adaptive psychological functioning. *Journal of Research in Personality, 41*, 139–154.
Newton, N. J., Herr, J. M., Pollack, J. I., & McAdams, D. P. (2014). Selfless or selfish? Generativity and narcissism as components of legacy. *Journal of Adult Development, 21*, 59–68.
Nunn, B. V. (2005). Getting clear what hope is. In J. A. Eliott (Ed.), *Interdisciplinary perspectives on hope* (pp. 63–77). New York: Nova Science Publishers.
Ojala, M. (2012). Regulating worry, promoting hope: How do children, adolescents, and young adults cope with climate change? *International Journal of Environmental & Science Education, 7*, 537–561.
Orne, M. T. (1968). On the nature of effective hope. *International Journal of Psychiatry, 5*, 403–410.
Ortony, A., Clore, G. L., & Collins, A. (1988). *The cognitive structure of emotion*. New York: Cambridge University Press.
Oveis, C., Horberg, E. J., & Keltner, D. (2010). Compassion, pride, and social intuitions of self-other similarity. *Journal of Personality and Social Psychology, 98*, 618–630.
Park, N., Peterson, C., & Seligman, M. (2004). Strengths of character and well-being. *Journal of Social and Clinical Psychology, 23*, 603–619.
Parker-Oliver, D. (2002). Redefining hope for the terminally ill. *American Journal of Hospice & Palliative Care, 19*, 115–120.
Persson, L., Lundegard, I., & Wickman, P.-O. (2011). Worry becomes hope in education for sustainable development. *Ultbildning & Demokrati, 20*, 123–144.
Peterson, C., Ruch, W., Beerman, U., Park, N., & Seligman, M. E. P. (2007). Strengths of character, orientations to happiness, and life satisfaction. *Journal of Positive Psychology, 2*, 149–156.
Peterson, C., & Seligman, M. E. P. (2004). *Character Strengths and Virtues: A Handbook and Classification*. Washington, D.C.: APA Press and Oxford University Press.
Pettit, P. (2004). Hope and its place in mind. *Annals of the American Academy of Political and Social Science, 592*, 152–165.
Post, S. G. (2013). Hope in caring for the deeply forgetful: Enduring selfhood and being open to surprises. *Bulletin of the Menninger Clinic, 77*, 349–368.
Quoidbach, J., Wood, A. M., & Hansenne, M. (2009). Back to the future: The effect of daily practice of mental time travel into the future on happiness and anxiety. *Journal of Positive Psychology, 3*, 349–355.
Redlich, D., Hadas-Lidor, N., Weiss, P., & Amirav, I. (2010). Mediated learning experience intervention increases hope of family members coping with a relative with severe mental illness. *Community Mental Health Journal, 46*, 409–415.
Reed, P. (2008). Theory of self-transcendence. In M. J. Smith & P. Liehr (Eds.), *Middle range theory for nursing* (pp. 105–129). New York: Springer.
Roseman, I. J., Spindel, M. S., & Jose, P. E. (1990). Appraisals of emotion-eliciting events: Testing a theory of discrete emotions. *Journal of Personality and Social Psychology, 59*, 899–915.

Schneider, S. (2001). In search of realistic optimism: Meaning, knowledge, and warm fuzziness. *American Psychologist, 56*, 250–263.
Schutta, K., & Burnett, C. B. (2000). Factors that influence a patient's decision toparticipate in a phase I cancer clinical trial. *Oncology Nursing Forum, 27*, 1435–1438.
Seligman, M. E. P. (1991). *Learned optimism*. New York: Knopf.
Singer, P. (1981). *The expanding circle: Ethics, evolution, and moral progress*. Princeton, NJ: Princeton University Press.
Snyder, C. R. (2002). Hope theory: Rainbows in the mind. *Psychological Inquiry, 13*, 1047–1084.
Snyder, C. R. (2004). Hope and the other strengths: Lessons from *Animal Farm*. *Journal of Social and Clinical Psychology, 23*, 624–627.
Snyder, C. R., Ilardi, S. S., Cheavens, J., Michael, S. T., Yamhure, L., & Sympson, S. (2000). The role of hope in cognitive-behavior therapies. *Cognitive Therapy and Research, 24*, 747–762.
Snyder, C. R., Rand, K. L., King, E. A., Feldman, D. B., & Woodward, J. T. (2002). "False" hope. *Journal of Clinical Psychology, 58*, 1003–1022.
Snyder, C. R., Sympson, S. C., Ybasco, F. C., Borders, T. F., Babyak, M. A., & Higgins, R. L. (1996). Development and validation of the State Hope Scale. *Journal of Personality and Social Psychology, 70*, 321–335.
Son, J., & Wilson, J. (2012). Volunteer work and hedonic, eudemonic, and social well-being. *Sociological Forum, 27*, 658–681.
Spencer, J., Davidson, H., & White, V. (1997). Helping clients develop hopes for the future. *American Journal of Occupational Therapy, 51*, 191–198.
Tesser, A. (1988). Toward a self-evaluation maintenance model of social behavior. In L. Berkowitz (Ed.), *Advances in Experimental Social Psychology* (Vol. 21, pp. 181–227). New York: Academic Press.
Thoits, P. A., & Hewitt, L. N. (2001). Volunteer work and well-being. *Journal of Health and Social Behavior, 42*, 115–131.
van den Bos, K., & Lind, E. A. (2001). The psychology of own versus others' treatment: Self-oriented and other-oriented effects on perceptions of procedural justice. *Personality and Social Psychology Bulletin, 27*, 1324–1333.
Wallmark, E., Safarzadeh, K., Daukantaite, D., & Maddux, R. E. (2013). Promoting altruism through meditation: An 8-week randomized controlled pilot study. *Mindfulness, 4*, 223–234.
Waterman, A. S. (1993). Two conceptions of happiness: Contrasts of personal expressiveness (eudaimonia) and hedonic enjoyment. *Journal of Personality and Social Psychology, 64*, 678–691.
Weis, R., & Speridakos, E. C. (2011). A meta-analysis of hope enhancement strategies in clinical and community settings. *Psychology of Well-Being: Theory, Research, and Practice, 1*, 5.
Wetherell, M., Taylor, S., & Yates, S. J. (2001). *Discourse as data: A guide for analysis*. Thousand Oaks, CA: Sage.
White, M., & Epston, D. (1990). *Narrative means to therapeutic ends*. New York: Norton & Company.
Williams, J. C., & Lynn, S. J. (2010). Acceptance: An historical and conceptual review. *Imagination, Cognition, & Personality, 30*, 5–56.
Williams, M. J. (2014). Serving the self from the seat of power: Goals and threats predict leaders' self-interested behavior. *Journal of Management, 40*, 1365–1395.
Wong, M. G., & Heriot, S. A. (2007). Vicarious futurity in autism and childhood dementia. *Journal of Autism and Developmental Disorders, 37*, 1833–1841.
Wood, A. M., Froh, J. J., & Geraghty, A. W. A. (2010). Gratitude and well-being: A review and theoretical integration. *Clinical Psychology Review, 30*, 890–905.
Yalom, I. D. (1998). *The Yalom reader*. New York: Basic Books.
Yalom, I. D., & Leszcz, M. (2005). *The theory and practice of group psychotherapy* (5th ed.). New York: Basic Books.

13543525R00070

Printed in Great Britain
by Amazon.co.uk, Ltd.,
Marston Gate.